Learning to Lead in the

Jeffrey L. Houpt • Roderick W. Gilkey
Susan H. Ehringhaus

Learning to Lead in the Academic Medical Center

A Practical Guide

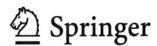 Springer

Jeffrey L. Houpt, MD
Dean Emeritus, University of North
  Carolina School of Medicine
CEO, Emeritus, University of North
  Carolina Health Care System
Chapel Hill, NC, USA

Susan H. Ehringhaus, JD
Senior Manager, Office for Interactions
  with Industry
Partners HealthCare
Boston, MA, USA

Roderick W. Gilkey, PhD
Professor in the Practice of Organization
  & Management
Goizueta Business School
Professor of Psychiatry and Behavioral
  Sciences
Emory University School of Medicine
Atlanta, GA, USA

ISBN 978-3-319-21259-3   ISBN 978-3-319-21260-9   (eBook)
DOI 10.1007/978-3-319-21260-9

Library of Congress Control Number: 2015946606

Springer Cham Heidelberg New York Dordrecht London
© Springer International Publishing Switzerland 2015

Printed on acid-free paper

Springer International Publishing AG Switzerland is part of Springer Science+Business Media (www.springer.com)

Foreword: Leadership Really Matters

If there is one thing that is evident from my more than 100 visits to academic health centers in the USA and around the world, it is the importance of leadership. I have seen leaders succeed and fail—and many who struggle. As I have gotten to know a good portion of them on a personal level, I have learned a lot about leadership skills as well as the process that brought them to leadership positions. Because academic health centers are complex institutions facing a highly challenging environment, with big budgets and many moving parts—not to mention egos—a high level of leadership skill is required. The necessary skill sets for these positions are usually discussed in broad general terms, such as "has vision," "is a good communicator," "works well with others," and so forth. But the tools to assess these characteristics, much less nurture them in potential leaders, are strikingly absent from the dialogue. More importantly, the key leadership attributes that involve personality factors, such as emotional intelligence, are even more rarely discussed.

What's needed is a handbook for current and aspiring leaders—hence the importance and relevance of this book. Houpt, Gilkey, and Ehringhaus do an extraordinary job of presenting both a broad overview of the dynamics of the academic health center and a granular "how to" for the myriad of situations that demand skilled leadership. This volume is abundantly filled with meaningful examples and worthy insights.

It is not surprising that in the world of academic health centers most leaders come from the academic ranks. This is both fitting and just, in that a deep-seated understanding of and respect for the core ethos of academia is indeed essential. Many such leaders are accomplished researchers, department chairs, institute and program directors, or come from other specialty-focused positions. They often have served at a high level in specialty societies, edited journals in their field, and been appointed to NIH study sections. But an insight I have obtained through my visits and personal contacts with academic health center leadership is that academic skills do not necessarily translate into leadership skills (Fig. 1).

Intellectual achievement, of course, is critical for academic success, whether it be in the creation of new knowledge, the development of a new program, or insightful commentary. However, intellectual ability does not necessarily imply that the necessary leadership behavioral skills are present, such as emotional intelligence

Academic		**Leadership**
• Intellectual capacity	—⟍—	• Emotional intelligence
• Narrow knowledge base	—⟍—	• Broad range of interests
• Strong work ethic	————	• Strong work ethic
• Highly self-motivated	—⟍—	• Highly institution-motivated
• Gets individual results	—⟍—	• Gets institutional results
• Rises up the academic ladder	—⟍—	• Manages 360

Fig. 1 Academic skills versus leadership skills [1]

and the ability to negotiate, which are well defined in this book. Most academics develop a specific and necessarily narrow knowledge base as a requirement for deep expertise in a specialty or research area. Yet, the successful leader of an academic health center must cultivate broad interests to effectively manage the institution, such as the "non-academic" pursuits of human resource departments, budgeting cycles, and public relations. Academically successful individuals are generally highly self-motivated in that their achievements are judged by what they do to benefit their careers. However, leadership of an academic health center requires institutional motivation in the sense that success is institutional, not personal. Institutional leadership therefore demands institutional results, which are far more diffuse and more difficult to sharply define than markers of individual success. The successful academic rises up the promotional and reputation ladder, whereas the successful leader must learn to "manage 360°," being rewarded by the achievements of others. (Of course, a strong work ethic, an honest character, and sound judgment are essential in any position.) There is thus much to learn for an aspiring leader who comes from a traditional academic background, and this book presents an excellent platform.

The pathway to leadership of an academic health center generally follows the timeworn tradition of academe by largely relying on a "search committee" that seeks an accomplished academic achiever. It is not unusual, therefore, for individuals with successful academic careers to find themselves 1 day in the position of "accidental leader," whereby success in one's field is assumed to automatically translate into successful institutional leadership. Or, perhaps, talented faculty who might be outstanding leaders eschew leadership, referring to it dismissively as "the suits" who are "sitting on a pile of money and not giving me enough of it." The problem thus is threefold: leadership is often opaque and vague to the faculty; academic success, as previously pointed out, is not necessarily the ticket to leadership success; and the search process for leaders is often flawed.

The authors conclude the book with a discussion of the challenges in finding the right leaders. I agree with much of what they say. Finding the "right" leader for a given institution is indeed a significant challenge. The actual search process, to the applicants and others, often appears unfocused and somewhat diffuse. Search committees, instead of concentrating on specific leadership abilities, often find themselves looking for the Deus ex machine, generally in the form of a physician–scientist, who will lead them into the Promised Land. In compiling a handbook of best search practices [2], I have suggested a set of guiding principles and basic management strategies to increase the likelihood of a successful search.

In brief, leadership searches should be given the highest priority, and the institution must be cognizant of the extent to which the search reflects on the culture and reputation of the institution. In many cases that I've observed, the search has been delegated to a search committee that often consists of institutional leaders with their own agendas about what is best for the institution. The search committee's role must be clearly defined and differentiated from that of the decision maker, who ultimately determines the terms of the contract to be signed, and who must be fully engaged throughout the entire process. It is essential that a broad and diverse pool of candidates be considered, and that the search process be well organized, preferably into three distinct phases: pre-search, active, and on-boarding.

Houpt, Gilkey, and Ehringhaus meet a critical need with this book. While the book reads logically from start to finish, the reader may want to prioritize certain sections. After brushing up on how the academic health center functions in Part I, the reader might try to recall personal situations in the past involving interactions with academic health center leaders that may or may not have come out well. These situations, for example, could involve negotiation, conflict resolution, or simply running a good (or bad) meeting. By reading the relevant chapters through a personal lens, the important lessons of the book become meaningfully individualized and then go on to serve as a platform for reviewing the remaining sections of the book. (Of course, this is just a suggestion, and I'm sure many readers will simply read the chapters in order.) Another thought is for the reader to discuss the various management scenarios presented in the book with a mentor or others in a small group setting, if that is possible, to both gain a deeper understanding and to practice specific skills. But please keep in mind that this book is more than a manual: it should be viewed as a highly personal journey toward a deeper understanding of one's strengths and weaknesses, and how this journey can enable successful leadership.

Academic health centers face a number of significant challenges in the twenty-first century. These include, among others, significant disruption with new care delivery and payment mechanisms, scientific and technological advances, and continued patient empowerment. It should be obvious that skilled leadership is essential to weather this perfect storm. The key to success in this environment, I believe, is the leader's ability to align the various missions (education, research, and patient care) so as to have each support and inform the others. Ultimately, the successful leader will be able to do so by changing culture and behavior. This book is a good place to start the journey.

Washington, DC, USA   Steven A. Wartman, M.D., Ph.D., M.A.C.P.
                                                 Association of Academic Health Centers

References

1. Wartman SA. Future shock or future success? The transformation of academic health centers: meeting the challenges of healthcare's changing landscape. Elsevier; 2015.
2. Wartman SA. Searching for leadership. Washington, DC: Association of Academic Health Centers; 2014.

Introduction

We always wanted to know what's in a book before we decide to invest the time to read it. And we thought you would, too, so here you are.

There are five parts to this book. The first three parts are narrative which are intended to help you learn to be a better leader. The first part looks at the AMC as a social system; the second at the role of personality; and the third at a set of necessary skill sets. The fourth part is a series of case vignettes to solve based on the material in sections which preceded it. The final part provides a set of solutions to those cases.

Part I attempts to take the mystery out of how the academic medical center (AMC) works. It can be intimidating to the novice leader with its size, built-in conflicts, and pressures to meet financial goals. Further, if the new leader begins, as many do, with a belief that its only control mechanisms are formal vertical hierarchies (dean to chair to division head), he or she is destined to play with one hand tied behind his or her back. Many novice leaders recruited from outside an institution compound the dilemma by mistakenly believing that what worked at their old institution will work at the new one. The reality is different. Each AMC has its own unique culture with its own control mechanisms that the leader needs to adapt to and actively use.

We suggest that you begin by looking at the AMC as a group—nothing more and nothing less—and by focusing on how a group functions. If you can understand how a group maintains control with both formal and informal mechanisms, how it clings to its values, why it rewards some and punishes others, how there are different interests within the same group, how and why the group bestows authority on its leader, and what the group wants from its leader, you are equipped to make decisions and to lead the organization to new heights. If, however, you veer off this pathway and violate deeply ingrained cultural norms, you will not be successful until you address these forces. Unfortunately, many new leaders have no awareness of these powerful forces.

The first part of the book provides ways to understand these issues, which we have framed in terms of group dynamics. The same dynamics occur for a dean (albeit on a more complicated level), chair, division head, training director, ward chief, and so on, and the lessons are the same. Our argument is that if you understand the organization's culture along with its power and authority structures, you've got important practical strategies for success as a leader.

The second part of the book takes up personality and its role in leadership. We cover the research on traits associated with leadership as well as the role of emotional intelligence. We also include a chapter on dealing with personality disorders. Biographical studies of great leaders suggest that many different types of personalities can be successful leaders. There is good reason to believe that success is a matter of "fit," that is, having a match between the individuals' characteristics and the requirements of historical context.

There is a large literature correlating leadership with certain personality traits, such as extraversion, to name just one. We review the traits that are most frequently associated with leadership, address how they may play out in the AMC, and offer strategies for compensating for weaknesses. Successful people compensate for weaknesses and play to their strengths. We extend this discussion by taking up the problem of managing personality-disordered people in the workplace.

In the final chapter of this part, we take up some of the most critical emotional intelligences. Their absence can be highly limiting or even major reasons for failure. We offer some suggestions for becoming better at these intelligences.

Thus the first two parts address the most serious deficiencies we see in failed or at least less than effective leadership: the inability to read culture and personality and emotional intelligence shortcomings. We believe that you can become a much better leader if you can learn how to use culture and to compensate for your personality shortcomings. But even if you can't, you can still learn to be a better leader by learning some basic management skills, which are the subject of Part III.

Part III begins with a chapter entitled "Getting Started." We believe the first year is critical to success. In this chapter we offer a way to apply the material outlined in the first two parts to your first year as a new leader and to avoid frequent rookie mistakes. Next we take up Negotiation and we outline a method of negotiating that is appropriate to the AMC. Since you will often be negotiating "up," where you have little or no power and where you must keep that person's good favor, you must be able to maintain relationships while negotiating. The most fundamental skill in negotiation is understanding the other parties' interests. This skill is also the foundation for the topics covered in the remaining chapters in this part—Recruitment, Conflict Resolution, Persuasion, Making Good Decisions, and Stimulating Change.

In Recruitment, we suggest that current methods often unfortunately breed conflict and adversity. However, if you base your recruiting methods on solid principles of negotiation, you can establish a spirit of cooperation and solidify positive relationships. Conflict Resolution is another type of negotiation that is also based on an understanding of interests. It need not be anxiety provoking. We use case vignettes to illustrate how you can build on your understanding of interests by incorporating concepts of personality and culture. Because of the nature of authority in the AMC, the ability to persuade is an all-important skill if you want to get anything accomplished. How much easier life is when you face nodding heads as opposed to angry rebuttals and threats. Like Recruitment and Conflict Resolution, Chap. 11 on Persuasion starts with an understanding of interests but also factors in the lessons on culture, the role of the leader, and personality.

Since groups are the favored means of doing business in the AMC, we add a chapter on Running a Meeting because the best-intentioned plans can be undermined by a group getting out of control. The role of the group leader is paramount in keeping the group on task, yet new leaders often have no experience in running groups or mental pictures of what they should be doing. We offer a method for understanding such a group and keeping it on task.

Making Good Decisions builds on Persuasion and Conflict Resolution and attempts to show how good decisions follow an algorithm that includes personality and politics. Good decisions also require timing or have tempo. They need not be too fast or impulsive nor too slow and conflict adverse. We also offer lessons learned from a lifetime of making decisions in the AMC.

Chapter 14 on Stimulating Change brings together the previous chapters' lessons and addresses how to change an organization without experiencing a coup. Stimulating change is the highest skill of the leader and requires incorporating all the lessons from this book.

The final chapter in Part III suggests simply that you can save an organization a lot of turmoil and enhance its chances for success if you pick the right person the first time. The chapter speaks to aspiring candidates about what they might want to be thinking about to ensure picking the right position. It also addresses what search committees should be considering in their own work.

Instead of focusing principally on examining CVs, which don't reveal whether someone has emotional intelligence, the important questions are whether the person can stand before a group and change how it thinks; whether he or she shows respect for all viewpoints; and whether the individual is prepared to go to a new psychological level where caring about the organization takes precedence over self-interest and pleasure is received from others doing well. We ask aspiring candidates to look at a possible job with an awareness of the skills it requires and to consider whether it fits their skill set and their stage in their own maturational cycle.

In Part IV, we offer nine cases and open-ended questions for reflection and discussion, all of which build on the lessons in Parts I–III. In Part V, we offer the same cases but with the addition of the answers and perspectives we suggest, based on our experiences in AMCs and especially our experience in teaching what's in this book.

This book was written to assist those rising to leadership positions in the AMC by shortening the learning curve. It can be used in two ways. First, as an individual you can read it as it is presented. Start at the beginning and read through the first three parts. Then, read the case vignettes in Part IV and try to solve them. And finally, compare your solutions to our solutions in Part V. Alternatively, for those in the AMC who wish to use this book in a class on leadership development, you could assign the first three parts as pre-readings. Then assign a case vignette or two from Part IV per session, and solve them as class exercises. As the teacher or discussion leader, you can use our solutions in Part V as a basis for teaching, or you can distribute our solutions after the class to compare with the thoughts of the class members.

We are often asked for additional references from the business literature that are relevant to what we cover in this book. We have collected those references in Appendix C.

Finally, we offer a note about the authors: this book reflects the experience of three authors, and generally, the views expressed are shared among all three. But many of the points made in the book are enriched by the perspective only gained through service as a leader within the AMC, rather than service in some other capacity in the AMC. These thoughts are uniquely those of Jeff Houpt. For ease of identification, we've indented these personal perspectives so that you can recognize the views and stories that could only have been gleaned from experiencing the AMC as first a faculty member, then a department chair, and then a dean and finally the CEO of a health system.

That's what is in the book. We hope you enjoy it.

Contents

Part II The Role of Personality

About the Authors

Jeffrey L. Houpt, M.D., is Professor of Psychiatry at the University of North Carolina, Dean Emeritus of the UNC School of Medicine, and CEO Emeritus of the UNC Health Care System.

He attended Baylor College of Medicine, interned in medicine at Boston City Hospital, and completed his psychiatry training at Yale. After serving at the US Naval Hospital in Oakland, CA, and the Pacific Medical Center, in San Francisco, he accepted a faculty position at Duke Medical Center where his clinical, research, and teaching interests examined the interface of psychiatry and medicine.

In 1985, he left Duke to become the Chair of Psychiatry at Emory University School of Medicine. There he developed new programs to address the field's growing emphasis in biology and neuroscience. After 5 years, the school selected him to be their dean. During his tenure, research funding doubled, new space was constructed, and the School of Public Health was launched from the School of Medicine's Department of Epidemiology.

In 1996, Dr. Houpt was named Dean of the School of Medicine and Vice Chancellor for Medical Affairs at UNC. With his leadership, the UNC Health Care System was created through legislation bringing together the hospitals and the faculty practice plan; Rex Healthcare, the premiere private hospital in Raleigh was purchased; a new genetics department and the Carolina Center for Genome Sciences were created; and the biomedical engineering department was expanded to be a joint program with North Carolina State University. Two new research buildings and an office building were constructed, and a new cancer hospital and adjoining faculty office building were in planning.

Since stepping down as Dean and CEO at UNC in 2004, Dr. Houpt has led a program in leadership development at UNC, been an executive coach and consulted to a number of medical schools, and chaired the Blue Cross-Blue Shield North Carolina Board.

He has served as President of the American College of Psychiatrists and the American Association of Academic Psychiatry. He has authored or co-authored 71 journal articles and edited 4 books, including the Importance of Mental Health Services to General Health Care (Ballinger Publishing, 1978) and Consultation and Liaison Psychiatry (Basic Books, 1987).

Roderick W. Gilkey, Ph.D., holds a joint appointment at Emory University, where he serves on the faculty of the Goizueta Business School as Professor in the Practice of Organization and Management and the School of Medicine, where he is a Professor of Psychiatry and Behavioral Sciences. Rick has also served on the faculty of Duke Corporate Education and as an Affiliate Professor at HEC Paris, France, in Executive Education.

Rick earned his graduate degrees at Harvard University and the University of Michigan. Prior to joining Emory, Rick was at Dartmouth College, where he held a joint appointment at the Amos Tuck School of Business and Dartmouth Medical School. Rick has served as a visiting professor of international negotiation at Groupe HEC, Paris, and as a visiting professor at INSEAD, Fontainebleau, where he has taught leadership and organizational behavior.

His current research is in the area of neuro-imaging, which involves the use of fMRI scanning technology to gain images of executives who are involved in strategic thinking, moral reasoning, and creative problem solving. This research is focused on understanding how the brain operates in the high level cognitive tasks with an executive population, and how to facilitate these types of learning and thinking.

Rick Gilkey's articles have appeared in several leading professional journals including The Harvard Business Review, and he has served as an editorial consultant to The New York Times and Fortune Magazine. Rick is co-author of a book on post-merger management entitled Joining Forces: Creating and Managing Successful Mergers and Acquisitions (Prentice-Hall), and he is a contributing author to Organizations on the Couch: Psychoanalytic Approaches to Understanding Organizational Dynamics (Jossey Bass). He is also editor and contributing author of The 21st Century Healthcare Leader (Jossey Bass). His most recent paper, "Using the Whole Brain to Think Strategically," (Gilkey, Cadeda, Bate, Robertson, and Kilts) in the Neuroleadership Journal was awarded the 2012 Paper of the Year.

Rick has provided consulting and executive education service to a broad array of corporations and non-profit organizations in the USA, Europe, and the Middle East, including GE, Citi Bank, Morgan Stanley, Carrefour S.A., SunTrust, Total AG, the Taskforce on Global Health, and the U.S. Department of State.

Susan H. Ehringhaus, J.D., is Senior Manager, Office for Interactions with Industry, at Partners HealthCare in Boston, MA. Before joining Partners in November 2009, she was Senior Director and Regulatory Counsel and Associate General Counsel at the Association of American Medical Colleges (AAMC) in Washington, D.C. from 2003 to 2009. While in Washington, she also served as Adjunct Professor of Law at Georgetown University Law Center. Prior to joining the AAMC, she was Vice Chancellor and General Counsel at The University of North Carolina at Chapel Hill, where she served as UNC's chief legal counsel for 29 years, as well as Adjunct Professor of Law at UNC's Law School.

She has been throughout her career actively involved in legal and policy matters relating to higher education and academic medicine, including issues in research, ethics, and integrity in academic institutions, technology transfer, conflicts of interest, health care, finance, business, and corporate affiliations. At Partners, her work focuses on interactions with industry across the Partners HealthCare system. At the AAMC her work involved regulatory, bioethical, and business issues in academic medicine and emphasized interactions with industry. As Adjunct Professor of Law, she taught the law of higher education at The University of North Carolina School of Law for many years as well as other courses, and while in Washington she also taught the law of higher education at Georgetown University Law Center.

The drafter of numerous institutional policies on various matters relating to academic medical center governance and ethics, she has served as an invited speaker and lecturer both nationally and internationally, as an author of papers on conflicts of interest and ethics in academic medicine, and as a consultant to many organizations on various topics relating to issues in academic medicine and higher education. She is the recipient of several honors and awards.

Part I
The Academic Medical Center (AMC): How It Really Works

Being an expert anthropologist is far more important to being a successful leader of an AMC than being an expert scientist or an individual highly skilled in finance. The skill set that gets you the job of a dean or chair includes your skill as a scientist, clinician, or teacher, but you will need an additional set of skills to lead. This additional skill set begins with understanding how this group of faculty, staff, and students who comprise the AMC is organized, what motivates them, who they listen to, and what they believe but may not share with you. The humbling fact is that they were a formed society when you arrived as leader and will be one when you leave. They already have their own rules, beliefs, and assumptions. To lead you must first catch up with them and figure out what they already know. That's what this first part is about.

Chapter 1
The AMC: The Formal and Informal Organization

The AMC

The Academic Medical Center (AMC), which we define as a medical school and its teaching hospitals, has an enormous impact on society and the nation's health. The Association of American Medical Colleges (AAMC) counts 141 US medical schools and nearly 400 major teaching hospitals as its members [1]. While they account for 5 % of all US hospitals, they provide 37 % of all charity care in this country. They provide the lion's share of specialty care: 100 % of comprehensive cancer centers, 68 % of all burn units, 78 % of level 1 trauma beds, and 59 % of all pediatric intensive care beds.

A large part of our nation's workforce for physicians is produced there, the majority of nurses and allied health professionals train there, and a large number of biomedical PhD's are educated there. 128,000 faculty, 83,000 medical students, and 110,000 residents work there every day [1].

Many Nobel Prize winners in medicine and physiology were trained there and work there. New treatments and technologies are tested and birthed there. Total research expenditures in 2011 for just the medical schools and teaching hospitals were $44.9 billion and generated 300,000 full-time, mostly highly skilled jobs [2].

The total economic impact from looking at all missions, teaching, research, clinical care, and community outreach, is staggering. Again, according to the AAMC, our nation's medical schools and teaching hospitals had an economic impact in 2011 of $587 billion and employed 3.5 million people [2].

Yet for all the might and power of these institutions, finding superior leadership is problematic. This has been especially true in the last two decades when a broader spectrum of skills has been demanded to manage the collision between the culture of academia and market pressures.

Because these institutions play such a pivotal role in the nation's health, and in the local and national economy, the stakes are high. Recovery from ineffective leadership can take years, and repeated transitions can paralyze these institutions.

© Springer International Publishing Switzerland 2015
J.L. Houpt et al., *Learning to Lead in the Academic Medical Center*,
DOI 10.1007/978-3-319-21260-9_1

The challenges to effective leadership are multiple. First, successful leadership requires bringing the two core institutions—the medical school and the teaching hospital—together in a mutually supportive way. Medical schools and teaching hospitals frequently have different governing boards with differing aims and criteria for choosing officers. Even in those cases where the hospital and medical school have common boards and officers, a cultural gap often remains between the business commitments of the hospital and academic commitments of the medical school/ university. In addition, the faculty practice plan is often a separate entity with different goals that are not always complementary.

Second, these enterprises are huge and have large leadership teams, requiring a level of coordination that is hard to achieve. In the case of the medical school, the leadership team is comprised of a dean, sometimes a vice president for medical or health affairs, 20 some department chairs, maybe ten center directors (interdisciplinary units), and anywhere from 5 to 20 division heads in each department, plus a series of associate and assistant deans for education, research, clinical care, faculty affairs, diversity, and other purposes at times. With the hospital, there may be 10–20 vice presidents and service line directors. Thus, one can have easily 75 people or so at the top whose activities need to be coordinated and who have to work collaboratively.

Third, unlike most businesses with targeted outcomes, products, and services, the missions for the AMC are different and multiple, including education, teaching, research, patient care, and community outreach, with outputs that are difficult to assess in either qualitative or quantitative terms. These different missions compete for resources and are often in conflict. For businesses, there is a financial profile that speaks for itself. In the AMC, a robust financial bottom line may actually indicate poor performance because it may have been achieved by skimping on mission-related activities, for example, education, in order to bolster the financial picture. Even defining a bottom line is a judgment call in the AMC.

Fourth, these organizations have multiple and independent levels of authority. The hospital likely has clear lines of authority—one for social work, one for nursing, one for materials management, etc.—thus leaving the physician, whose line of authority is back to his or her department chair, to fend for himself or herself with each separate discipline with which he or she comes in contact. Further, with an AMC leadership team of 75 or more, accountability can often be elusive.

Fifth, all of the units are interdependent. Operating room efficiency doesn't improve unless all parties pull together—physicians, nurses, orderlies, pharmacies, those who clean the rooms, and more. As an added complication, some clinical programs are profitable, and others are not. Cross subsidies must be a way of life. Unlike businesses, unprofitable business lines cannot be eliminated. Pediatricians are essential, but they rarely are profitable service lines.

But profitability as a concept is more complicated than simply looking at one service line. In an AMC, the more profitable service lines are often downstream. The downstream radiologist is profitable, but only if the pediatrician who requires a subsidy is in place.

However, the biggest problem is that the skill set that makes for success in academia and thus makes one a candidate for a leadership position is not the same skill set that makes one a successful leader of a large, complex enterprise. Despite the necessary attention given to working effectively in a team context, especially in medicine, success in climbing the academic ladder still requires originality of thought and independence in the discovery of new knowledge. It's still based on independence and being a strong individual contributor. You are evaluated on your own demonstrated and documented work product. It takes persistent pursuit of ideas and the ability to compete with peers in order to secure resources. Being a successful leader, however, requires a different skill set. A leader must look out for the group's interest, not his or her own, and the skill set that is required must include listening, persuading, acting in the face of conflict, understanding the nuances of culture, managing interpersonal conflict, having a confident demeanor, and being interpersonally sensitive. This is a set of skills that is viewed as soft. Only an astute search committee finds an overlap of both skill sets. Many search committees continue to pursue academic all-stars with little interest or aptitude in leading a group.

Should these challenges lead to despair or desperation? It need not. Happily, people can learn to traverse this troubled terrain. These massive entities with their myriad challenges need not intimidate you. The challenges produce conflicts complicated by human eccentricities, but you can learn how to deal with them. We can't eradicate the hardwired aspects of personality that stand behind an individual's lack of emotional intelligence, but we can mitigate and manage them. We can try to eliminate the bad habits that emanate from them. And we can exploit strong points and add new skills that will make everyone—naturally gifted or not—better. That's what this book is about. But this understanding all begins with giving you simplified mental schemas with which to understand what looks like a hopelessly conflicted and complicated field. If you understand what governs behavior, you can manage the organization, despite its complexity, and lead it in new directions.

Simplified Mental Schemas

Initially, think of the AMC as a group—nothing more and nothing less. The primary function of a group is to survive. Hence, the first task of the leader is to convince the group that you can and will help them survive.

And think of the faculty member as seeking to do whatever is in his or her best interest. He or she wants you, as the leader, to be maximally effective in assisting in carrying out his or her work. She needs to see you having that interest. The clinician wants readily accessible radiology and laboratory services, beds when needed, accurate billing, etc. The researcher wants decent lab space, top-of-the line core facilities, an efficient grants office, etc. The educator wants respect and compensation. These expectations should be easy to grasp; it's all the things you wanted when you were in one or more of those positions.

The first lesson to learn as a new leader is that you are not there to tell the faculty what to do, but to convince them that your purpose is to enable them to survive and prosper. In other words, you must gain credibility to lead, and to do so, your first task as the leader is to convince the group that you will help them survive. Only then can you speak to higher goals and aspirations. Following a Maslow-like hierarchy, if the members of the group feel secure, that is, their job is not in jeopardy and the compensation is reasonably intact, they move with a sense of urgency to higher-level tasks. They become concerned about the trajectory of their career, their national standing—individually and as a group (division, department, school, hospital, healthcare system).

History proves this point. All groups have a division of labor and have developed rules that they live by to ensure that they can live peacefully while surviving and prospering. One of the earliest divisions of labor was between the hunters and the gatherers. Life was simple. You hunted or you gathered. However, with the discovery of tools, and the transition to an agrarian society, there were excesses of production, and with excesses came commerce, and with commerce came money, and with money came questions about how to divvy it up. As resources expanded, new groups incorporated tools, and they became capable of competing more effectively, and with competition came the need to expand markets.

Different roles were developed, e.g., landowner, laborer, merchant, and banker, and with different roles came the development of hierarchies: landowner/laborer, head banker/teller, and shop owner/clerk. Work or effort was translated into money. Haves and have-nots emerged. To maintain order, groups embraced and created culture, that is, the rules of what is fair and what is acceptable behavior and what is not. Some of the rules were spoken and others not, possibly out of fear of retribution. Leaders emerged who either represented the group's culture and interests or not.

A ruling class emerged. While the Fertile Crescent created the world's first society based on above-subsistence agriculture, it also created the first caste of organizational leaders as the priests of Samaria ascended to power. Coups were staged against "bad" leaders, i.e., those who did not represent the group's interests or were carried away by greed. But, in each case, informal organizations were formed on the basis of cultural values, whether formally acknowledged or not.

AMCs are not that different from these early groups; they possess the same governing systems, some reflecting control and management and others reflecting culture. These systems are also motivating systems, and they perform both functions effectively.

The Three Governing Systems

There are just three governing/motivating systems within the AMC. First, there is the hierarchical system or formal organization. In the medical school, the governing system refers to the dean, chair, and division head and in the hospital, the president, vice presidents, and so forth. The second is the compensation system that directs behavior by what it rewards. And the third is the informal organization, a product of the culture. The informal organization is a web of values, mores, and mental representations or archetypes with its own set of leaders that guide the faculty and staff within the AMC with regard to what is right and wrong and what is respected and what is not. Some of these values and archetypes are overt and talked about, while others are beyond day-to-day awareness but ever so determinative of behavior. These are the unspoken values and web of beliefs that many novice leaders are oblivious to. Failure to recognize them accounts more often for a leader's failure or ineffectiveness than any other reason.

Most people in leadership positions in AMCs understand the first two governing systems, but new leaders often overestimate their utility. Said a different way, they don't understand the limitations of these two systems, and they limit their effectiveness by relying exclusively on them. In so doing, they totally miss the informal organization, a critical component of the governance of the AMC. We will return to this concept throughout this book, because it is essential to recognize and utilize the power and influence that come from gaining credibility in this domain.

Hierarchical Systems

The most important impact of the hierarchical system is that it can get you hired or fired. It also sets your compensation within the constructs of the university and its policies.

Hierarchical systems are useful for establishing quality standards. The chair and division head's job is to set standards for performance within each discipline. Standards are the means for recruitment of the best and finest. They inform the entire organization on expectations for the field, and their responsibility is to ensure that those expectations are met.

However, a focus on hierarchal systems breeds insularity and excessive attention to vertical communication. This in turn leads to maintenance of the status quo and lack of coordination, and survival/supremacy within areas or silos becomes the dominant motivation.

Hierarchy as a governing/motivating tool fails as a mechanism for working among groups or for reaching overall institutional goals because institutional goals may not be seen as being in the best interest of a particular group. In the face of mounting financial pressures, for example, this conflict between group goals and institutional goals becomes exacerbated.

Unfortunately, the naive often beat their head against the wall, relying repeatedly on hierarchical systems to accomplish trans-system goals.

Compensation and Other Resources

Likewise, compensation as a motivating system is effective, but only up to a point. Financial incentives are great when pursuing financial goals. Such incentives are relatively easy to understand and to conceptualize. But they often fail in supporting trans-system goals described above. More importantly, they miss what motivates faculty and thus fail to engage a powerful lever for harnessing and directing the energy of the faculty.

In a word, financial incentives don't speak to mission—the soulful or spiritual side of the equation. Faculty work not only for money but for the excitement of the intellectual challenge and for the quest to find a new scientific breakthrough or a new treatment. They work in a useful narcissistic bubble—they believe they can be the best in the world at what they do. They come to work excited because they think they might actually find an answer for diabetes or dementia. CEOs who create reward systems based entirely on money get what they want—a faculty only interested in money. Faculty subjected to such a world view soon figure out that if it is all about money, they prefer going into private practice or industry and making more money. Those who remain become obsessed with money and seek numerous ways to get more—usually by threatening to leave. Their institutions are constantly putting together retention packages, and there are constant struggles over resources. The missions are lost and the organization loses its soul.

Culture

What the champions of hierarchies and financial reward miss is the role of culture and, as an offshoot, the role of what we refer to as the informal organization. New leaders, as well as established, ineffective leaders, often ignore it—they don't even see it—and thus they fail. Every organization has invisible assumptions and values that underlie its visible behavioral norms, its artifacts (overt signs of the culture), and its performance (tangible results). Culture has to be understood as comprising both the visible and invisible; it is the context in which a leader succeeds or fails.

One dimension of culture is the "informal organization," that is, the "village elders" whose opinion perfectly reflects visible and invisible norms and artifacts. They are the true leaders of the group. They are not necessarily those leaders placed within the vertical hierarchy, but they often have some administrative portfolio. For example, a division head in medicine may be a village elder but the chair may not be. In the informal organization, a village elder does not derive his or her authority from the chair but has authority independent of the chair. The individual has authority only because his or her opinion is listened to and followed. There is no formal election; the village elder is just the de facto leader. The village elder's influence is amplified because there is a constituency of people, a bloc of votes, behind him or her.

There is no way to lead an AMC with just two governance systems, hierarchy and finance. Only by navigating and using the culture and the informal organization can you mitigate the complexities of the AMC, overcome its conflicts, and assist its people in choosing solutions that are not always in their own financial self-interest.

It is the most powerful of all the governing or motivating systems. It is so important, and so often missed, that the next chapter, Culture is King, deals with norms, artifacts, and archetypes in greater detail. Then Chap. 3, Authority Is Earned, extends the discussion of the informal organization.

However, one more factor is needed on how groups function in order to utilize these three levers: how information flows in the AMC and the consequences for the new dean or chair.

The Creative Society Versus the Efficient Society

If you want an efficient operation, you want information to flow top down. You want everyone knowing their role and following it to the letter. Many businesses in the 1950s, 1960s, and 1970s embodied this model. Imagine an automobile manufacturing company. The R and D section is loaded with engineers that decide the specifications of new models—aerodynamics, stress, gas usage, aesthetics, etc.—and then decisions are made at the top and they move to production. Workers are expected to be in lockstep. This permits maximal efficiency and embodies the efficient society. This model has been the cartoon dream of old-school hospital directors. But the upside potential for innovation and improvement is limited because it empowers a limited population that lacks diversity.

However, the medical school has traditionally valued creativity and innovation over efficiency. Faculty have been committed to the creative/innovative society. To the faculty of the medical school, the entire school is an R and D tank, with a heavy emphasis on R. In such a society, information has to flow multidirectionally—from the bottom up, from the top down, and horizontally and diagonally too. The greatest level of specialization and those closest to the cutting edge, and thus those who have the most knowledge, are on the bottom; the ones with the broadest view but with the least specialized information are on the top.

The people who know the latest on science and what needs to be invested in are on the bottom: the ones who make the financial decisions of what to invest in are on the top. The clinicians who know the specifics of what needs to be changed to improve quality are on the bottom, while the ones who know the least about this but who control the decisions and finances are at the top. This dislocation of specialized information and decision-making creates conflicts daily in the AMC, particularly as margins become narrower. New deans or chairs who begin with a proclamation "we are doing this (in the interest of efficiency)" are met with "wait, I know more about this than you." And so it goes. The hospital director thinks he or she knows best, or the dean thinks he or she does and they force a top-down model. Meanwhile, the faculty doesn't just think they know best, they know what's best. This is one aspect of culture missed by many deans and hospital directors.

This decoupling of the best information from decision-making often causes great consternation among new deans. They are unsure what to do when they are not the thought experts. They all came through the same system and hierarchy. As division chiefs they knew their field and were thought leaders. As chairs, depending on the size of the department, they also were thought leaders, at least for part of the department, but when they are deans, they are not the experts.

> For example, I as a psychiatrist had to make significant decisions about genetics. There was no way that I could do that based on my knowledge of genetics. I had to get the information from the experts (at the bottom of the hierarchy). And then I had to prioritize it against other requests, say in surgery – again in a specialized field I was not an expert in.

Some cannot make this transition. You have to go from being a thought expert to being the person who asks the right questions and has the right advisors around to make good decisions. Rejoining information with decision-making requires multi-directional information flow. The point is that you can't succeed without information flow from the bottom.

But you also cannot succeed if there is no information flow from the top to the bottom. By being at the top, you have broader vision and more information, though it is less detailed. You need to set priorities and determine and articulate a vision. The vision has to be seen as enhancing their success and survival. Only when you do that can the people in the trenches of the organization understand and buy-in to your decisions.

Summary

The AMC is a group and as such it wants to survive and prosper. Once its more basic needs are met, they are replaced with a growing list of aspirations. There is never a sated state. Until the leader convinces the group that he or she can help them survive and help them achieve broader goals, the individual will not be given the authority he or she needs to be their leader.

Embedded within the group are a series of governing mechanisms that were in place long before you became a leader. There are vertical hierarchies, compensation systems, and the culture, both spoken and unspoken, that provide an informal organization. The mechanisms and organizations are there for your use. Hierarchies and compensation systems have strengths and weaknesses; use them wisely. The sleeper of the group is culture—it can help you accomplish what hierarchies and compensation systems can't. If you learn how to use and leverage it, you can become a transformational leader.

It's not that complicated, at least in theory. How you apply it is more complex and takes practice, but that's what this book addresses.

References

1. American Association of Medical Colleges [Internet]. Washington, DC © 1995–2015. Available from: https://www.aamc.org/about/membership/378788/medicalschools.html
2. Association of American Medical Colleges. The economic impact of AAMC-member medical schools and teaching hospitals. Washington, DC: AAMC; 2012.

Chapter 2
Culture Is King

A new dean addresses the faculty in her annual faculty meeting. She speaks about medicine being a business and in the course of this discussion indicates that "we need to be more responsive to our customers." When she offers time for discussion at the end, an esteemed senior faculty member stands up and says, "I have patients, not customers." Six months later, most of the faculty have decided that the dean "doesn't get it." Her many initiatives go nowhere, as they are stymied by passive–aggressive faculty behavior.

xxxxxxxxxxxxxxxxxxxxxxxxxxxxxxxxxxxxxxxxxxxxxxxxxxxxxxxxxxxx

A junior faculty member on a yearly renewable contract is not renewed after four years when the chair decides that he is not likely to secure research funding. He files a grievance, and a committee finds that the faculty member was not sufficiently mentored and reverses the chair's decision. The chair is aghast because he followed the steps outlined by the university attorney.

xxxxxxxxxxxxxxxxxxxxxxxxxxxxxxxxxxxxxxxxxxxxxxxxxxxxxxxxxxxx

The head of the faculty practice organization asks its budget committee to review the subsidies to the departments of family medicine and psychiatry. The committee unexpectedly recommends abandoning all subsidies. This puts a total of six departments in the red and reverses twenty years of precedents.

xxxxxxxxxxxxxxxxxxxxxxxxxxxxxxxxxxxxxxxxxxxxxxxxxxxxxxxxxxxx

What do all of these vignettes have in common? They represent decisions made that are not in the best interests of the institution. And they all represent initiatives whose outcomes could have been avoided. They all were initiated by principals who failed to appreciate the importance of culture and could have been avoided by leaders who understood culture.

© Springer International Publishing Switzerland 2015
J.L. Houpt et al., *Learning to Lead in the Academic Medical Center*,
DOI 10.1007/978-3-319-21260-9_2

Culture Is King

Edgar Schein, the esteemed professor at the MIT Sloan School of Management, proposed that organizational culture could be viewed at three different levels; first, artifacts including the visible elements of an organization, e.g., dress code, architecture, etc.; second, espoused values or public statements; and, third, shared basic assumptions or deeply embedded, taken-for-granted behaviors that are often unconscious [1].

Culture creates the context in which leadership succeeds or fails. Culture includes values or norms and archetypes (mental representations). Values and norms as well as archetypes operate at both a conscious and unconscious level. At an unconscious level, they are particularly powerful. Together they are the algorithm by which we process information to decide what's good, or permissible, and what is not. They also provide us with an idealized image of what we should be.

From the point of view of leadership, an understanding of culture can be useful in four ways. First, you can use culture to define differences between schools. Culture gives the school its personality. There's an old adage: "if you've seen one medical school you've seen one medical school." It's the respective culture of each medical school that distinguishes it from others. To take a job at a new school and not understand its distinct personality is akin to entering into a long-term relationship on the basis of appearances without understanding the other person's beliefs, proclivities, sore spots, loves, and longings. Yet it's done all the time with predictably negative results.

Second, you can use your knowledge of culture to better understand conflicts between faculty members or between departments or between factions within departments. Faculty holding different norms and archetypes will come to different conclusions when presented with the same data. Similarly, departments or factions within departments with different norms or archetypes will come to different conclusions with the same data.

It's true that the predominant culture accounts for each school's personality, but cultural differences among people exist as well. This accounts for why committee decisions depend almost entirely on the composition of the committee, as illustrated by the decision of the finance committee of the faculty practice organization, and the story of the junior faculty member above.

Third, understanding culture is necessary to carry out any change agenda. Change is initially almost always resisted. The easiest way to create an unhappy opposition is to violate a commonly held value or cultural norm. As an example, to enter a school that values processes, that is, the faculty's role in governance, and then to make pronouncements simply won't work. In addition to values being the prompt for resistance, holding a different unspoken archetype can also form the basis for a person to resist.

Finally, the faculty determine their willingness to permit you to lead based on their assessment, at least in part, of whether they believe you represent their values. Knowledge of the culture or ignorance or a violation of it typecasts a leader as a fit or misfit. Once people say, "he just doesn't get it," your power and reach are severely limited. Alternatively, "she's got the right values" is an accolade that permits you to take on difficult and intransigent issues. Clearly, the new dean in the example at the beginning of this chapter didn't get it.

> Faculty who are about to take on larger administrative jobs often believe their biggest short-coming will be their lack of knowledge of finance. It's not. Faculty often come to me to discuss if they should take a certain job. When I explore their insecurities and concerns, inexperience in handling finances is often what they are most anxious about. It's under-standable, but misguided. What's far more important is the ability to read the culture. It's much better to be a good anthropologist than a whiz at finances. You can delegate the finances. You can't delegate an understanding of culture. Your every action demonstrates your understanding, or lack thereof. The remainder of this chapter speaks to how to become a better anthropologist.

Values and Cultural Norms: Distinguishing Between Schools

> I'm not aware of any studies of values and norms in AMCs or any that yield a typology. My work experience has permitted me to see three schools intensively, while my coaching experience has given me an opportunity to see several additional schools "up close and personal." I've become convinced that there are a recurring set of values that drive behavior and decisions, and by clustering them together, you can distinguish one school from another. I have no tests of reliability or validity, nor can I pretend that this is a complete set. But when presented to my coaching clients as a way to think about their school, they find it useful. It gives us a common vocabulary to begin mapping the keys to their culture.
>
> I propose that schools can be distinguished by where they fall along a continuum from one pole to another along a set of dichotomous variables.
>
> These variables are:

COMMON VALUES FOR SCHOOLS OF MEDICINE

Process/Executive Control
the degree to which the organization requires faculty approval versus allows leader initi-ated activities

Ranking and Honors/Mission
the value the institution places on rankings versus on meeting its mission

Individual Stars/Equity
the value the faculty place on outstanding scholars even when they consume excessive resources versus an ideal that resources should be evenly distributed

Care and Feeding/Darwinism
the degree to which an organization feels that an individual faculty member needs assis-tance to succeed versus the survival of the fittest, that is, the feeling that the strong will survive and that survival is a useful sorting mechanism

COMMON VALUES FOR HEALTH SYSTEMS

Remunerative/Comprehensive services
the balance between profitable services and loss leaders

Cost Containment/Faculty Desires and Needs
how much margin is fed back into programs?

Efficiency/Teaching and Research
the tolerance for education and research when it creates inefficiencies

Gain-sharing/Central Control of Resources
are margins distributed by formula or held centrally requiring all to go "hat in hand"?

Cross-subsidy/"Tub on its own bottom"
the willingness to cost shift

Try out your own school and place it with these variables and values. I can distinguish UNC from Duke and Emory, I think, on these dichotomous variables. UNC would favor process over executive control, mission over ranking, equity over stars, and care and feeding over Darwinism. Duke and Emory would tend to be in the other direction. My co-authors have formed similar impressions, from different vantage points.

We believe that these are relative distinctions. Take process and executive control. We've already stated that the most strongly held value in academia is the freedom to pursue ideas without constraint. But within that value there are differences in degrees of freedom. In some schools, that sentiment is extended to the belief that faculty have a primary role in decisions of governance. In those schools, process—how decisions are made and specifically that faculty have a say—is strongly embraced. In fact, the process of how decisions are made can be more important than what decision is made, up to a point. In other more "executive" schools, there is a sense that faculty should be consulted but the final decision belongs to the administrative head, e.g., dean or chair. What is decided is valued more than how it was decided.

In the process value schools, there is a sense that faculty councils should take stands on academic issues and that faculty meetings should provide an opportunity for comment. Committees are used liberally, and few major policy decisions go forward without beginning in committee.

In those institutions favoring executive control, the sense is that the dean or chair hasn't come of age until he or she takes ownership of an important issue. This involves a public statement or commitment to an initiative that will succeed or fail (i.e., has risks) that all are aware of.

In executive control schools, faculty councils limit their range of interest to generic issues, that is, sabbaticals, more scholarships, or debating admissions policies. Committees are used sparingly and are viewed as a waste of time by many faculty. Faculty meetings are used to praise the accomplishments of the faculty; they are not viewed as useful settings to make decisions. Of course, these values are not mutually exclusive. These are tendencies, not absolutes, but organizational preferences or default positions reflect the organization's culture.

Values and Norms: Differences Within Faculty of the Same School

Recall the example of the junior faculty member who was given a notice of nonrenewal. The chair tells him that he will not be renewed. He files a grievance, for example, on the basis of discrimination, and a committee hears his grievance. Listen to one set of questions from one committee member, a care and feeding type: (1) Were you given a mentor? (2) Did you get feedback about how you were doing? (3) Were you given adequate release time? (4) Did the chair give you warning that you would be let go if you didn't get funding this year?

But a Darwinian committee member may ask a different set of questions: (1) Did you seek feedback? (2) What did you think would happen if you didn't get funding? (3) Why didn't you ask the chair what you should do? (4) Why would you think you'd be subsidized forever?

These sets of questions clearly show the difference between care and feeding faculty and Darwinians. In the end, the decision on this faculty member will be determined to a large degree, if not entirely, based on a set of values. In the example presented, the care and feeding types predominated and formed a majority of the committee.

This example makes an important point about committees: their decisions will depend to a large degree on their membership, especially in areas of disagreement among faculty. Since we use committees so broadly, this point is of utmost importance.

> This is why faculty who can suspend their personal bias and look to the good of the institution are so critical. As dean, I had a mental scorecard of who could rise above bias and who couldn't, and who could look to the interests of the institution rather than just their own and their department. I could not use some otherwise very good people because of their bias and their absolutely predictable behavior patterns.

In addition to differences among faculty, there are also differences between departments.

> We have a second home on one of the San Juan Islands in Washington. It has microclimates, which is to say that the sun can be shining on one part of the island, and it can be raining on another part. Academic medical centers have cultural microclimates or subcultures, which complicate the task of leadership enormously.

Each department tends to evaluate itself against a national reference group. The department of pediatrics does not compare itself to the medicine department in its home school but to other pediatrics departments across the country. Orthopedics compares itself to other orthopedics departments, psychiatry to psychiatry, and, for large medicine departments, individual divisions (e.g., gastrointestinal, cardiology, infectious diseases) to their national counterparts.

So there are at least 30 cultural microclimates, each with its own set of inborn ideas of excellence, fairness, hierarchies of status, beliefs with regard to autonomy, and so forth. This allegiance to national norms plays out most dramatically in concepts of tenure. Based on a national reference point, the orthopedic department will have a vastly different perspective on the qualifications for tenure, for example, from the department of medicine. No matter how the dean parses it, the sun will shine on one part of the kingdom, and it will be raining in another, and the same is true for the chair with his or her division heads.

Sometimes a part of one department aligns itself more closely with the values of another department than with its own department, putting the chair in the same bind that the dean often faces. In the clinical departments, this is most easily seen between the cognitive specialties and the procedural.

The proceduralists in cardiology, for example, may align with their surgical colleagues, while the geriatricians, the cognitive specialists, align with the psychiatrists and pediatricians. The cognitive specialists may favor subsidy, whereas the proceduralist may favor "each tub on its own bottom." No matter how the chair parses it, the sun will be out in one part of the kingdom, and it will be raining in another.

Values and Norms: Critical to a Strategy for a Change Agenda

Every attempt at change is either consonant or dissonant with an existing value or norm. Attempt something that's consonant with an existing value, and it's likely to be accepted. It's called "low hanging fruit." Violate an embedded value and an initiative will be resisted. Call it a "third rail issue."

Never undertake any change agenda without anticipating how it will be viewed from the standpoint of cherished values. Getting faculty to move beyond perceived value clashes is a key skill of the transformational leader. Anticipating the reaction of others requires using your empathy to foresee how others will feel about the proposed change. In this context what you think about the proposed change is less important than how others are likely to feel about it.

The dean cited in the beginning of this chapter appeared to violate the norm of the institution, which was cryptically noted by the esteemed senior faculty member.

We used the words "senior" and "esteemed" to describe the faculty member who challenged the dean as a means to signal that he filled a role as village elder. This means that when he speaks, people listen. He is a thought leader in the institution imbued with authority from the informal organization. You should always try to enlist the village elders to your side when embarking on change. This harnesses the power of the informal organization, that is, the organization's cultural levers that are not dependent on hierarchies. An enlightened dean would have immediately realized that an aspect of the informal organization had been revealed and would have called him to arrange a face-to-face meeting, not to criticize him but to find out exactly what he meant by his comment that he had "patients, not customers."

Let's assume we did talk to him, and we learned that he is concerned about the increasing commoditization of medicine. He notes a decline in the commitment to the classical model of the doctor–patient relationship, and he thinks that business speak only secularizes what he sees as an almost spiritual bond. Further, he believes that the trouble with the practice of medicine today is that physicians are compelled by challenges associated with the changes broadly in healthcare to see patients as numbers with particular conditions to be addressed, not as unique complex beings in the classical model. All the new dean's talk about healthcare being a business and her talk of clients only confirmed that this new dean did not get it and was part of the problem and was the wrong person to be leading the institution.

Had the dean talked to this faculty member, the discussion could have gone in two different ways. The dean might have agreed with the sentiments of the faculty member and reformulated her message about "customers" as referring only to a new commitment to amenity, efficiency, and service, but not as an attack on the doctor–patient relationship. Or she might hold the value that medicine is a business that has historically been practiced poorly and needs the help of successful business models. In the first case, the dean would be salvaged; in the latter the judgment of the dean as not getting it would be upheld. In either case, the values of the dean and their compatibility with the informal organization would be laid bare.

Values and Norms: Determining If the New Leader Is a Fit or a Misfit

Equally important as understanding the values of the organization you are being asked to lead is understanding your own values. To be successful, there needs to be a fit.

Kouzes and Posner argue that the first commitment that the leader needs to make to his or her constituents is to clarify his or her values. They argue that there needs to be a fit between the values of the institution and one's own personal values. They cite research that finds that success occurs in those instances where personal values coincide with institutional values [2].

> When I took my first job at Duke, my mentors said that it was a good fit. I never asked them what they meant other than to realize that they thought it was a good choice. When I left Duke to go to Emory as chair of psychiatry, I thought that Emory was a good fit. By that I meant I thought its challenges matched my skill set.
>
> When I left Emory to come to UNC I thought that it was a good fit because I thought that my values and those of UNC were a good fit.
>
> Looking back I now realize that fit has two dimensions. One is a match of job requirements and your competencies, and the second is a shared set of values. Both are important. Problems ensue if either competencies or values are not a fit. Ideally you should have ferreted out the fit before you decided to take the job. Search committees should be looking for it as well.

The new dean mentioned above represents a conflict between her personal values and the predominant values held by those within the institution. Over a 6-month period, the faculty had come to agree with the senior clinician that the new dean was not the person to lead the institution. Conflicts over values, often barely formulated into words or discussed, hold powerful sway. She just didn't get it.

Core Values: The "Super Values" that Trump Others

Within any group there are values that are sacrosanct or at least said to be. In Schein's model [1] they fall into category two, the spoken values. The group rarely goes against them publicly. To align yourself with them will usually allow you to win your point. To violate them, in the absence of a large campaign to redefine them, usually means that you lose the point. They trump other values that are not viewed as core.

However, do not assume that if you drape yourself in them, you will always win the day. While publicly espoused, these values may not be universally accepted. Sometimes they conflict with personal gain, and sometimes they conflict with other core values, in which case they don't prevail. You need to listen and watch responses to discover the real acceptance of these values, notwithstanding their public prominence. Some examples follow:

1. Excellence: to demonstrate that a proposed course of action will extend the excellence of a program in many places means that we "must do it-end of story." To wrap your proposal in that flag ensures immediate acceptance, you would think. The problem is that the commitment to "excellence" is often only given lip service. Excellence is great if it means that the resources are going to you instead of others.

> As an example, I know a very senior person who is an honored and esteemed investigator who, one would assume, would embrace excellence across the board but who exploded with, "Any money that goes to someone else and doesn't go to me is wasted!" Decisions based on excellence have also been torpedoed on the basis of unfairness or inequity, or on the fear of bringing in people viewed as boorish.

Nevertheless, it is a powerful core value. To be a dean or chair and to embrace it puts you on higher ground. While people may grumble and hold resentments, a commitment to excellence doesn't harm a person in leadership. You want to declare that this is what you are about. It should trump all political considerations. For a state-supported school, excellence is the way to ensure good stewardship of tax dollars or, in the case of private school, the best use of philanthropic funds.

2. Rankings: several schools have set about with the express purpose to improve their rankings. It's commonplace for prospective deans and university presidents to talk of improving their ranking. However, faculty do not always share the view of the dean and university president.

One can pretty easily determine if this is a super value by knowing whether the faculty easily buys into the idea of rankings as being a legitimate goal of the university or school or, if on the contrary, there is a lot of discussion about whether the rankings are a reliable guide to quality and relevant. Opposition to rankings as a core value can be focused on claims that they reflect only the size and past reputation of the faculty and not current quality or that they don't honor a particular mission.

While you might want to embrace excellence as a core value, despite some who find reason to oppose it, espousing rankings is much more complicated because of the disagreement over the metrics to define ranks. If you go down that road, you will likely have to defend your metrics. While excellence is just as hard to define, it is a more acceptable goal to pursue, whereas rankings immediately bring the US News and World report rankings, NIH rankings, and other rankings into the debate.

3. Mission: this is especially important to some state-supported schools and community-based schools. At UNC, the commitment to serve the people of the state is a core value. I was surprised when I first arrived as I had suspected that it might just be paid lip service.

> However, I did a Delphi survey, asking the faculty "what would UNC as a model medical school look like", only to find that commitment to mission trumped all other considerations. In community based schools, a commitment to serve the people in a particular region of the State and providing primary care physicians to that part of the state will drive much of their thinking.
>
> In other schools, the mission consists of a statement that is hung on the wall, and no one believes it has meaning. Just the thought of crafting a mission statement brings audible groans.

4. Collegiality: getting along civilly is a core value in some places. In such places, the ability to work collaboratively is highly valued. Norms exist that dampen emotional outbursts. The senior investigator who intoned that only his work should be funded would be viewed as an outcast. The collegial workplace is so valued that it is the major recruiting tool to bring in faculty, and a selection bias reinforces the value. However, these places face strains when this norm must be reevaluated when an outstanding candidate for faculty membership (a star) is self-centered, is hard edged, or is even mean in dealing with people. A decision needs to be made along the lines of: "can we get by with one of these?" Generally, a decision is made that there are other stars out there, who combine excellence with collegiality. In such cases, collegiality trumps excellence. In other institutions, their definition of excellence is a matter of counting up how many stars they have. In those places, hiring the star wins out.

Repeated decisions of collegiality over excellence can lead to mediocrity, whereas deciding for excellence over collegiality may lead to fiefdoms and poor morale or environments described as "eating their young."

5. Process: in some schools, particularly but not exclusively state schools, how decisions are made and who participates in them can be more important than what is decided. New programs are nonstarters without ample faculty input, whether through faculty committees or standing faculty councils.

Seemingly, simple no-brainers can ignite resistance. A basic science chair who suggests that all graduate students will need to be supported by grants is initially opposed vigorously within the school. A year and a half later, after full faculty discussion, the same group decides to unanimously adopt that position. In a second example, a new clinical chair begins an ambitious strategic planning process and hires a leading consulting firm to assist. Okay? Not so fast. The faculty objects to the firm, but after a month's discussion they embrace the idea. Or the chair of the neurosurgery department attempts to institute a new compensation plan that more strongly rewards individual productivity over group achievement in hopes of recruiting more highly paid specialists. The department objects to the change. One year later, following participation in the development of a new plan very similar to the original proposal, the faculty supports "their" plan, and the hires are made.

Archetypes

In addition to thinking about culture as a set of values and norms, a second way to view culture is to ask the questions: "How do faculty really think their society should be organized?" "Do faculty have the same conception of the ideal society, and if not, how do their conceptions differ?"

> A number of experiences have led me to the idea that some faculty had a preconceived notion of how their world should be. As we traversed the managed care years of the 90's, there was a real sense of mourning and loss, especially from the older faculty members, about the pressures for efficiency and the movement to metrics to measure everything they did. There was a longing to return to how things were. They felt a great loss of autonomy and a sense that this was not the world that they signed up for. Arguments that things had changed and the institution needed to move on were understood on a conscious level, but resisted intra-psychically. I remember doing my best to adapt to this new world, and to move the institution forward, only to have several faculty severely disappointed that I wasn't fighting it – as if in their omnipotent fantasies of me, I could turn managed care back to usual and customary charges.
>
> A number of years later I was coaching the chair of a large, research-intensive department when he forwarded an email to me from one of his faculty members.
>
> In it the faculty member complained that he, the chair, didn't understand that his role was not to micromanage but to stand back and support the faculty in what they did, like the Medicis did. He should finance and support them, praise them and appreciate them.
>
> The mention of the Medicis, coupled with the mourning of the loss of autonomy, brought this together for me. The faculty was mourning the loss of the medieval university. They had an archetype in mind, a mental representation, of how the ideal academic society should be constituted. Their disappointment with me was that we weren't doing enough to sustain it, and, in effect, were permitting it to slip away.

In the medieval university archetype, the faculty believe that they should enjoy unfettered freedom and that whatever they do is great and should be supported. This includes a guarantee of a job, a salary, and a space. Tenure is the defining concept.

In the current world, those who hold this view are scrupulous with regard to who holds tenure. It's only for the elite. Accordingly, there may be disdain for clinical track faculty and a bold line can be drawn between tenure track and research track basic science faculty. There's an emphasis on independence. There is no "deadwood" among the tenured faculty. They prefer to see unfunded but tenured research faculty as "post-award," that is, a legitimate developmental landing place.

In short, there is no reason, financial, political, or otherwise, that should undermine the full meaning of tenure.

Support for this view may be more prevalent among long-term faculty who were trained in this model. But it also finds expression in some of the more influential writings of our day. Ludmerer, in his highly acclaimed book, *A Time to Heal*, complains about clinical faculty "who have no attributes of faculty," of deans who go to Washington to seek funding for research (presumably instead of trying to change the world back to the way it was), and the return to "proprietary" schools concerned only about the bottom line financially [3].

We would call the second archetype that has emerged the technological/entrepreneurial model. Here, faculty are committed to solving a problem—a big problem— whether it is diabetes, cancer, or a basic science problem like how the genome functions. These groups tend to operate in multidisciplinary fashion and are organized in highly focused teams.

A core value for them is efficiency. For them, the work is serious and there is no messing around. Also, excellence is absolutely essential. This is a team effort, and the team is only as strong as its weakest link. And here is where they diverge from the medieval archetype. There is no room on the team for anything less than excellence and lacking funding definitively defines the absence of excellence.

"Post-award" faculty should be treated nicely but have their salaries trimmed and space taken away. In the best of all worlds, unfunded faculty should assume a larger teaching role, freeing up others to do their groundbreaking research or take on jobs running core facilities or, better yet, just go away voluntarily. For them, what's important is the research product. They believe in tenure with regard to academic freedom, but not as long-term salary guarantees. Salaries available from faculty who voluntarily retire (as they should when unfunded) should be put back into the big problem they are working on. Salary should be based on productivity.

Elements of this model find expression in Thorp and Goldstein's book, *Engines of Innovation: The Entrepreneurial University in the Twenty-First Century* [4]. Here the measure is not just student, research, and clinical performance but also the number of patents and number of innovations that have improved the world or the health of the people.

Interestingly, while this model is compatible with current financial pressures, it didn't emerge for financial reasons. Rather it grew on both clinical and research sides of the campus when independently the faculty concluded that doing their best work required teamwork. This sentiment was driven home for me when at UNC, when one of our leading investigators was lured from the university to set up in nearby Research Triangle Park by an investor. The investor wanted him to focus on his research full-time, hoping that it would lead to a cure for a disease that the investor had a personal interest in.

In the end, the investigator decide against it, not because of any counter offer, but because he concluded that while his work required physicists today, it might require mathematicians tomorrow, and another group the next day. He realized that research was a team sport and that there just wasn't enough money to recreate the university elsewhere.

The same is just as true on the clinical side. Cancer treatment is multidisciplinary, diabetes treatment requires case management, and psychiatric treatment needs psychosocial rehabilitation and family education. You can't just go it alone and be excellent.

This model has great appeal as a way to deal with economic pressures and meet the obligation to society to reduce morbidity and the burden of disease. It replaces the felt loss of autonomy of the medieval university with the compelling passion to take on the big problems and make the world a better place. The ivory tower is no longer composed of people lost in their own idiosyncratic thoughts who were valued in the medieval society. Instead the value now is on getting together and doing something really useful and big.

However, to most faculty in this group, there need to be at least two modifications to make this model palatable. First, they need to be in an environment that places a high value on independence, and second, in a place with sufficient freedom for an individual to dream up important experiments for which there is presently no immediate application.

The third archetype is the economic/capitalistic model. It has been the intellectual home to many hospital directors for years, to the business people who occupy our boards of directors, and to deans and chairs in the last 10–15 years. It's relatively common with clinical faculty, especially those who practice clinically nearly full time. In this archetype, the idealized university permits and rewards people for their individual productivity. It gives license for faculty to act out of their own self-interest, in keeping with the basic rule of economics. The underlying belief is that behavior can be manipulated by aligning incentives. To this group, the ship can be moved by paying people more if they produce and less if they do not.

The role of the medical school, particularly the administration, is to clear the obstacles to their practice; turn the operating rooms over more quickly; always have rooms cleaned and available for their admissions; make those techs in the catheter lab stay there until the physicians are ready to go home, not at the end of their shift; have the pharmacy stocked at all times; find more pleasant staff in the clinics; etc. And, finally, if an individual's extra work improves the hospital's bottom line, share that with that individual.

To this group, tenure is often an anachronism. There should be none. Faculty should be paid for performance only. Clinical workhorses who generate dollars should be paid accordingly. There is no leeway for senior faculty who were clinical workhorses earlier in their career. Their pay drops as their productivity does. This is hard for them because when they were younger, they subsidized the older clinicians, like senior partners in a law firm who built the business. Now, the younger generation weaned on an economic model are no longer willing to do that.

Likewise, basic scientists or clinical investigators should be paid based on the number of grant dollars they secure. Deadwood exists and should be moved out. This archetype does not support cross subsidy. In the example provided at the start of this chapter, the faculty practice organization committee looked at family medicine and psychiatry subsidies and voted the economic/capitalistic model.

We end with a vignette, which is designed to show how archetypes can lead to misunderstanding and an inability to resolve conflict.

The dean's office has been working with the chair of a basic science department to trim his budget. According to the financial people in the dean's office, the department could trim $1.5M over three years by a series of decisions—letting an assistant professor in year 4 without funding go and cutting back the salaries of less productive senior faculty to university-approved base salaries for tenured faculty and by taking away their space and reassigning it to productive faculty.

The chair appears to agree but doesn't do it.

This could be understood a number of ways. One could view it as some in the dean's office did. They viewed him as conflict averse; others viewed him as passive–aggressive. Of course, psychiatric diagnoses are the greatest of ad hominem arguments. He's ignored and worked around, once he's "diagnosed."

On the other hand, he could be a devotee of the medieval university and truly dedicated to its precepts. In reality, the chair's discussions with the faculty suggest that. He's telling them that he is fighting for their academic freedom. He's hardly conflict averse or passive–aggressive, since he's fought openly with the dean's office before and with the provost.

Those of us who hold one model or another tend to be blind to the validity of any other model. This kind of egocentric bias is pervasive and leads to all kinds of conflicts and misunderstandings. In this situation, for example, the finance people in the dean's office embrace an economic model, and so they see the chair's behavior as inexplicable short of a psychiatric diagnosis.

The dean holds the technological/entrepreneurial model and so just gets irritated at the chair's unwillingness to embrace efficiency and get with the important business of solving the greater problems. The chair views the dean and her staff as devotees of the economic model and as "heathens at the gate," jeopardizing the future of the university. Accordingly, he is on his way to choosing a path of martyrdom and is about to create a war of principles, enlisting the faculty to support him.

As an alternative you could view him as a well-meaning person, without psychiatric diagnoses, with a medieval world view, and approach him accordingly. By understanding that he has a different world view, you approach him as sane. What people hate most is being treated as if they are idiots or psychiatric cases. And what sane-minded dean doesn't fear for the university in this commercially crazed world? Can't the dean convey her concern for commercial influences and still be reassuring that she will continue to champion the causes of the university, even though in this case she needs to rule against him on two points: one is on the basis of efficiency and, the second, on the basis of fairness. Since other chairs have gone through the process of reassigning space and altering salaries according to approved guidelines, so must he.

That dean doesn't need to convert him to her entrepreneurial model. She can genuinely express an understanding of where he comes from. And she can avoid ad hominem arguments. Everyone who disagrees with you does not deserve a psychiatric diagnosis. Being an anthropologist and understanding norms and archetypes can help you unlock conflicts and find areas of agreement.

To summarize this chapter, culture is king. It defines the school and it distinguishes one school from another. It also sets up conflict within schools. It determines the ease of successfully establishing new initiatives. And it speaks loudly to the success or failure of a leader because it requires a fit between personal values and institutional ones.

Successful leadership requires affirming core values. It requires negotiating disagreements when values conflict. It requires reaffirming values and redefining them in the current context. It requires understanding archetypes.

As I reflect on my time as dean, I now realize (I didn't then) that every major change initiative must include at its inception an understanding of culture. Whether it's negotiating with your president, attempting to bring two programs together in a single one, or purchasing a hospital and integrating services, all depend on defining underlying beliefs and assumptions and, when necessary, redefining them to meet new goals. Subsequent chapters will apply these concepts in more detail.

References

1. Schein E. Organizational culture and leadership. 4th ed. San Francisco: Jossey-Bass; 2010.
2. Kouzes J, Posner B. The leadership challenge. San Francisco: Jossey-Bass; 2007.
3. Ludmerer K. A time to heal. Oxford: Oxford University Press; 1999.
4. Thorp H, Goldstein B. Engines of innovation: the entrepreneurial university in the twenty-first century. Chapel Hill: University of North Carolina Press; 2010.

Chapter 3
Authority Is Earned, Not Bestowed

The new dean and the president are in the president's office enjoying time together shortly after the president has appointed the new dean. Together they talk excitedly about their goals and aspirations for the medical school and the academic medical center. These celebratory conversations anticipating great glories are common across the USA. They occur in about five to fifteen places each year, marking the turnover rate of deans, and the topics are similar: moving the school into the top ten, creating the area's best cardiovascular center and thus stabilizing the finances of the hospital, and so forth. If there is any discussion of what it's going to take to achieve these goals, it's limited to a number of positions and space. There's no discussion of culture or of authority, let alone an implementation plan or how to handle collateral damage.

Shortly thereafter, the enthused new dean calls a faculty meeting and announces his "charge" from the president—that is, the dean's and the president's vision. For reasons that are never clear to the dean, the faculty resists his initiatives and after a short term of two or three years, the president who was the architect of this plan fires him. The collateral damage isn't a cost the president wants to bear. The story need not turn out that way.

In another AMC on the very same day, assume the following was taking place.

*The new dean begins her first day by having breakfast with the president who hired her. She always enjoys her time with him. They've shared their mutual expectations for the academic medical center. They're in lockstep in their thinking. But unlike the dean noted above, she doesn't wish to start out by telling the faculty what will happen. She's thinking: "He's so rushed. So impatient – maybe he had ADD as a kid. Doesn't he get it? This idea of his that people have bought into the translational center…Sure they think it's a good idea now, but we've not even considered what we **can't** do if we put our money there. Sure we can do it, but then we can't do something else. He doesn't seem to understand the need for buy-in or the trade-offs, which haven't even been considered. I've been around a bit and one thing I know: People always resist change. They always fear that they are going to lose something.*

© Springer International Publishing Switzerland 2015

J.L. Houpt et al., *Learning to Lead in the Academic Medical Center,*
DOI 10.1007/978-3-319-21260-9_3

Even if it looks good to them, they resist. Further, there must be reasons they haven't done it before. No, I'm going to do this my way...I need to get some things done first. I've got to build trust. I've got to meet face to face with the constituents – faculty, staff, alumni, hospital people and so forth. I've got to get some good will in the bank...and I need to get some buy-in from the leaders. It's a decent idea but it's not fleshed out yet. It's not yet ready for prime time."

If you are taking on a leadership position in the AMC, get used to the fact that it's not only what you do but also how you go about doing it. The best ideas will be left on the drawing room floor if you don't know how to navigate the culture of the AMC. And that knowledge begins with an understanding of the nature of authority.

In an earlier chapter, we commented on the limited value of vertical hierarchies. A most unfortunate and damaging expression of that notion is that new deans or chairs rarely have the authority to act on whatever charge has been given by the person who hired them, whether the president, the dean, or even the search committee. What they don't realize is that all the president can bestow on the dean is the title. The president cannot bestow authority. Likewise, the dean can bestow the title of chair, but not authority.

Authority can only grow out of the leader–constituent interaction. It has to be earned. The dean's authority is bestowed by his or her constituents—the faculty primarily, but also the chairs, the president, alumni, trustees, and others important to the institution. For chairs, only the departmental faculty can bestow authority.

John Gardner was president of the Carnegie Corporation and the Carnegie Foundation for the Advancement of Teaching (1955–1965), US Secretary of Health, Education, and Welfare (1965–1968), and founding chairman of Common Cause (1970–1977). In his book, *On Leadership*, he says the leader–constituent interaction is "the heart of the matter...." "Leaders are almost never in charge as they are pictured to be" (p. 23), and "Leadership is conferred by followers...." "Executives are given subordinates; they have to earn the followers" (p. 24) [1].

This concept follows from the discussion in the first chapter on the AMC. The first purpose of the group is to survive, and its second is to thrive in a way it defines. The leader must first convince the group that he or she is that person who is committed to their survival and thriving. That's a two-step evaluation: (1) Does the individual have our interests at heart, and (2) can the individual deliver success? Question #1 is answered in the first 6 months, or 12 months at most. Question #2 takes longer.

We suggested earlier that the faculty know more than you because they have the greater specialty knowledge. They also have an advantage over you especially if you are recruited from outside the organization. Because they've been around longer, they have mastered the informal organization. They can simply outlive you and resist you. They will be there when you leave.

As one faculty member confided in me once when talking about their new but already unpopular dean, "Oh we can outlast him. We've had bad deans before."

I recall having to decide whether to take the chair's position at Emory. The dean who sent me the offer letter abruptly resigned to go to another institution, and I had to decide whether to go into the situation without a permanent dean. I called Dean Warren, the chair of surgery there. He had impressed me when I interviewed there. He had been a dean at another institution previously, and had resumed his career as surgery chair at Emory. He was affectionately called Dean, or Dean x 2 and he was the leading village elder. His response was totally unexpected, but has caused me to chuckle many times. *"You come on down here. Let me tell you how it works. A good dean recruits the 23 smartest individuals he can find to be chair, who then spend all their energy deceiving him. There is no dean we can't get around. So don't you worry."*

New deans and chairs need to accept this: they are no match for the collective intelligence of the faculty and their ability to read culture and work the informal organization, which is either for or against you. You either work with them, or they work against you.

Our dean #1 missed that—the entire schema of how the AMC really works. No, they didn't welcome his announcement on his first day of what they were going to do. Who is this arrogant man?

We're not advocating for deans or chairs who don't have ideas. Nor are we suggesting a democratic vote on everything. Nearly as damning as not asking their opinion is the conclusion by faculty that the new dean or chair has no ideas. In a place where good ideas are valued above all else, you must have ideas. How you include the faculty in the development of your ideas is what's important.

Our dean #2 above knew all this. She understood what buy-in meant, that choices to fund one thing meant not doing other things (which inevitably meant that some faculty in that audience would correctly conclude that they were not the priority), and that she had to earn her authority.

It's all in how you do it. This sounds so easy but it is not. Here's how it happens. The new leader begins with a list of all the things that need fixing, which of course is read as all the things that are wrong with the place. At an emotional level, the faculty hears that their baby is ugly! And, unfortunately, that's all the new leader says. So the faculty goes further in their thinking and concludes that the leader wants to kill their baby, which explains the strength of the emotional reactions a new leader can provoke.

Dean #1 should have just started with a comment like dean #2 did. She said: *"I'm excited to be here. I've long admired x, y, and z about this place. I wanted this position because I felt that we had similar goals and aspirations and would work well together. In listening to you in my interviews, and to the search committee, I heard some things we need to address – like a, b, and c. I will be using the next few months to get to know you and to get your input on what we should do and to find ways that we can address them."*

These comments make several points—we don't have to tear this place down; your baby is pretty; I like you; I share your values; I have ideas; I'm going to act; I'm going to consult with you; and we won't act until I hear from you. Most importantly, the comments are in keeping with the formal and informal organization.

This distinction we're drawing between authoritative and participatory systems is reflected in the business literature as well. There it is framed as command and control management versus learning organizations [2]. The prototypic control and command organization is the military. In the traditional view of the military, authority is directed from the top down through a set of commanding officers so that a specified action is accomplished.

In academia, a learning model like Senge's is a far more useful model for administration [2]. In this model, opinions are sought throughout the organization; debate, discourse, and dialogue are encouraged; and the group commits to mutual learning. The leader nurtures this process rather than dictates a direction.

Power Versus Earned Authority

Webster defines power in a couple of ways [3]. One is "physical might," which implies unquestioned strength and the ability to act with impunity. This is not what we are talking about here when we speak of authority. You do have some power as dean or chair. As we mentioned earlier when referencing vertical hierarchies, you have the power to hire, fire, and set salaries (within the confines of university policy). But earning authority is something very different. It happens when the faculty give you authority to act; they trust you to do so in their best interests. They want you to speak for them, and they trust that you will stand up for them. You may have the power to set salaries and hire and fire, but when you have earned authority, they want you to represent them.

Earning Authority Is an Emotional Process

This whole process of gaining trust or earning authority has a large emotional element. While there are cognitive elements to be sure, it is still decidedly an emotional leap of faith. I did a small, highly scientifically uncontrolled experiment, but its findings illuminate this process. I asked people I knew well already, some 6–12 months after they had gotten a new dean or chair, whether the person was "any good." For chairs, I asked faculty within the department; for deans, I asked faculty from any department.

Here's what I heard:

"He'll be okay. He listens."
"She's got a lot to learn, but I think we [faculty] are willing to teach her."
"He's very smart, but so tight, into himself."
"Has the right values."
"Impulsive, too quick to make decisions, never met a question he didn't have an answer for."
"He's a natural – we love him."
"So direct, so abrupt, so in your face."
"Surprised us – he consults widely."
"One of us – he'll be okay."
"No human juices, so boring, so stilted."
"Imperious, comes across as critical all the time."

Note that all the answers reflected whether the faculty were willing to bond to that person or not. True, the person may have been forced into early decisions, and so there are some cognitive elements that contribute to the assessment. But for the most part, the comments seemed to reflect a "sizing up" based on shared values, on being "teachable," and on consulting and respecting faculty. There is also a strong emotional element involved as people decide whether they feel sufficiently comfortable to trust and empower the new leader. From the comments, you can accurately predict which individuals being assessed would earn authority and which ones would not.

In our experience from coaching and watching leaders in chair or dean positions, they gain acceptance in the first year. If they do not earn authority in that time period, they have a difficult term.

Authority Is Only Bestowed When It's Approved by the Informal Organization

You will recall that the informal organization derives from the values, norms, and archetypes of the institutions. The informal organization also sustains the values, norms, and archetypes of the organization by "throwing out" anybody who violates them too severely. They do this by refusing to bestow authority.

> Culture is a set of ideas, whereas the informal organization is people. The most important group is the "village elders" as I have called them. They are the opinion leaders - the ones people listen to and choose as role models. Every organization has them; the leader's job is to find out who they are and cultivate them. When it comes to bestowing authority, they are the deciding vote. It is they who say, "Yeah, okay, I get it, she has some flaws, but she's okay. She's on our side - we can trust her."
>
> Shortly after becoming the dean I reviewed the MCAT scores (aptitude tests) of the entering medical students. I found that they were about at the 60th percentile, while the school is ranked in the top quartile on about every other conceivable measure. As might be expected, when I commented on this in a faculty meeting, it rankled the admissions committee and created a stir with the entire faculty. (Here I am saying that their baby was ugly.) In order to deal with the brouhaha, I went to the admissions committee and met with them, which lead to a healthy discussion about admission criteria. It also resulted in changing some members of the committee. In the end it settled down, but only after some personnel changes. There was no singing Kumbaya around a campfire. Some egos were bruised and remained so. I never knew why it died down and so one day after I had stepped down, I asked one of the committee members (a village elder) her view of what happened and why it settled down. *She said, "In the end we knew you had the school's interests at heart, you listened to us and made your case, and we decided you were okay."*

A second set of actors in the informal organization are the "mafia." These are powerful people outside the hierarchy who nevertheless have immediate access to the president or dean. They are donors, legislators, trustees, influential alumni, or local dignitaries. Their importance is great because they can pick up a phone and immediately get the ear and attention of the president and can call for an action to take place. They grant you authority with their peer group—the president, trustees, legislators, donors, and others. Gaining the support of that group goes a long way to being able to make transformative changes and to weathering attacks from within. We will talk more about gaining support in Chap. 14.

Authority Is Distributed

If the first rule is that authority has to be bestowed, the second rule is that it has to be shared or distributed.

In the case of the dean, authority is shared with at least three parties—with his or her immediate reports, for example, the vice and associate deans, the chairs and center directors, and the appropriate people from the hospital or healthcare system. For chairs, authority is shared with vice chairs, division heads, and appropriate people in the hospital/healthcare system.

For both deans and chairs, coordinated activities among all groups give the leaders the best chance of meeting their objectives, whether academic, clinical, or financial. Uncoordinated activities make those objectives unreachable. With coordinated activities, a sense of well-being and high morale pervade the workplace; with uncoordinated activities, fiefdoms and divisiveness develop. It is difficult to build relationships to members of these groups without this distribution of authority.

Consequently, a key task of leadership for a dean or chair is the creation of a well-functioning system for distributing authority. Success depends on the following parameters being met:

1. A consistent message, aligned with the vision/mission and a common set of values;
2. An implementation plan with objectives and time lines;
3. An easy exchange of ideas, with appropriate opportunities for disagreement and reformulation;
4. Tons of praise for a job well done.

Management of these relationships in which authority is shared is crucial to success for either a dean or a chair. From the dean's perspective, two deserve special attention: the relationship of dean to chair and dean to hospital/healthcare system. The relationship of dean to chair and dean to hospital director is reciprocal. Each person's success is enhanced with a committed and energized partner who can understand and focus on a common set of goals. And similarly, the success of either is compromised with an unwilling partner. You can't find a maximally successful dean without a supportive and committed medicine chair, a successful medicine chair without a committed dean, a successful hospital director without a supportive dean, or a successful dean without a partner in the hospital director. The success of each depends on the other.

And so it is in AMCs. Authority is earned, and just how that is accomplished will be taken up in Chap. 7. And authority is distributed. Everyone's success depends on others' success.

References

1. Gardner J. On leadership. New York: Free Press; 1990.
2. Senge P. The fifth discipline. New York: Doubleday; 1990.
3. Merriam-Webster Dictionary. Encyclopedia Britannica. www.merriamwebster.com/dictionary/power.

Part II
The Role of Personality

You might view the first part of this book as depicting the AMC as a social organization. This second part examines the individual personality traits and emotional competencies that are required to effectively lead that social organization.

Your personality is the vehicle through which you lead. While your cognitive capacities are the threshold competencies needed to get considered for the job, your personality and emotional attributes are the factors that enable you to be successful.

This part examines personality by considering traits and emotional intelligences. What traits and what emotional intelligences are needed, and do you have them? Is there a way to compensate for shortcomings and learn to overcome them? And because we open the subject of personality traits, we also take up how to manage personality disorders in the workplace.

Chapter 4
Personality Traits and Leadership

"Why bother, you can't change personality" *was the response of a distinguished colleague when told of our chapter on personality and leadership.*

"She's just wired right" *was the comment of a senior administrator when admiring the skill of a younger colleague in a leadership position.*

"He just can't make a decision" *commented a frustrated faculty member about the leader of his area.*

"I'm not ever going to pursue a chairmanship. I can't stand all the conflict… people fighting with each other over a finite set of resources" *complained one faculty member.*

"We're going to get the right person this time – someone who can help us rebuild morale and instill a sense of mission and purpose" *said a hopeful member of a search committee.*

These comments reflect some of the common conclusions about personality and leadership.

One view is that personality is hardwired. How many times have we heard that leaders are born, not made, or the adage "the cream always rises to the top" and that leadership can't be taught—that "he or she is a natural leader." We can argue each of these points, but the common belief is that personality is hardwired and determines leadership ability. So why bother even thinking about it if you can't do anything about it?

Another common view is that the decision of most people to pursue leadership positions is determined in large part on their own assessment of their personality. We know that some people who are extremely talented and intellectually capable do not wish to take on leadership positions. When questioned, their reasons are often based on features of their personality—too risk averse, conflict avoidant, publicity adverse, or intolerant of political and manipulative environments. And some avoid leadership positions because of the emotional stress they feel. On the other hand, we also know those who crave the spotlight and the feeling that comes from being the leader, despite having no interest in doing the job or with little

© Springer International Publishing Switzerland 2015
J.L. Houpt et al., *Learning to Lead in the Academic Medical Center*,
DOI 10.1007/978-3-319-21260-9_4

capacity to do so. They seek these jobs and get them, only to detest all of the work that comes with them.

A third common view is that dealing with people with personality disorders in the workplace is frustrating, emotionally depleting, and a major reason for burnout. Taken with the assumption that you can't change people, it is apparent why some throw up their arms, saying "it's impossible."

Still another view is that we can depend on the search process to screen for the attributes that we should be seeking in a leader. We continue to hold to the view that we can pick the right person, yet given the number of failures, there might be reason to question that optimism.

All these views reflect the crucial role of personality, but in negative, almost hopeless, ways. But what if you start out with a different set of assumptions? What if you affirm the important role of personality but allow for the possibility of compensating for weaknesses, so that you don't have to score a perfect ten on some imagined scorecard? What if you assume that no one is perfect and that the question is not whether you have what it takes but whether you have *enough* of the right stuff and can make yourself better? What if you could learn new skills that would make you not only more effective but also less emotionally depleted by doing these jobs?

We believe that a realistic assessment of your own personality is a critical piece of data, perhaps the most crucial piece, in deciding to undertake these jobs or not. Not everyone in academia should pursue these jobs; some should continue their clinical work, teaching, and research. We believe people should pursue areas where they can have the most positive influence. But you should decide on the basis of an informed opinion of personality and its role rather than on popularly held assumptions.

Further, what if there were strategies to deal with personality disorders in the workplace that limit their stress on us? We don't mean strategies to "fix" them but strategies to mitigate their effect on the group and also on you as the leader. And what if, based on a better understanding of personality, we could construct a better scorecard of what search committees should be looking for and thus pick better candidates?

We believe that we can make a case for these latter possibilities. In this chapter, we will focus on personality traits. We will attempt to do so by reviewing current concepts of leadership, based on biographical and psychometric methodologies. Having reviewed the findings, we will examine them against our knowledge of the AMC.

In Chap. 5 on Managing Personality Disorders in the Workplace, we will focus on the management of certain personality disorders and how their effect in the AMC might be mitigated. In Chap. 6 on The Importance of Emotional Intelligence, we will look at that concept as a different and useful way to view personality in leadership. We will specifically focus on three emotional intelligences—listening, other-centeredness, and demeanor. In all of these areas, the overriding aim will be to illustrate how you can improve whatever deficiencies you might have in these areas.

Biographical Approaches: What Biography Teaches Us About the Important Role of Context

Biographical studies have produced no single personality type that makes a leader successful but rather have found that the greatest leaders have experienced both failures and successes in their lives. This has shifted the focus from seeking the "one-size-fits-all" leader to understanding the person within his or her historical context.

The lives of Churchill and Lincoln both illustrate this latter view. Churchill had authored five books by age 26 and had escaped Boer prison camp before launching a successful legislative career. Named the Secretary of the Exchequer in the conservative Baldwin government, he returned Britain to the gold standard. When that maneuver had a deflationary effect, he was sent out of politics.

However, the context changed. As a result of World War II, Churchill was called on to be the First Lord of the Admiralty. When Neville Chamberlain resigned in May 1940, Churchill then became Prime Minister. Using his oratorical skills and his natural moxie, he became known as one of the greatest wartime leaders of all time. Many have surmised that Britain would not have survived the war without him. But he was dropped in a postwar election. One conclusion to draw is that historical context required a different kind of leader.

Lincoln's career also illustrates the importance of context. Lincoln failed at his first business, which was as co-owner in a grocery store, despite good economic times. He became a country lawyer and forged a state legislative career. He enjoyed a so-so career until slavery became an issue and he arose to the presidency. He became who many view as our best president.

Erik Erikson defined leadership as the perfect collision between the right historic moment and the right leader [1]. The "fit" we're talking about is probably not a passive fit, like placing a piece in a jigsaw puzzle. It is more likely an active process where the leader finds the wherewithal to adapt and meet the longings of a constituency at a historical point in time.

Thus, the aspiring leader should be asking himself or herself, "is this the right fit for me? Do the institution's needs fit with my skill set?" And search committees should wonder if this is the right person for this institution at this time. We see this focus on context in AMC searches as well. If you ask search committees what they are looking for, you will often uncover a characteristic that they think meets the "current" need. "This time we need someone with passion," if a quiet yet successful leader has just stepped down. Or if the leader had been charismatic and transformative, you will hear pleas for someone steady or level headed.

Psychometric Approaches: What the Big Five and Myers–Briggs Teach Us About Personality Traits

There is a rich research tradition that has tried to move beyond the subjectivity associated with anecdotal speculation. Over the past 50 years, psychologists have found reliable measures of personality and, armed with these tools, have studied their correlations with leaders. Of all the measures available, we will limit ourselves to just two: the Big Five [2] and the Myers–Briggs Inventory [3] because of their widespread acceptance.

The Big Five

Many have advanced the idea that personality is comprised of five basic dimensions. Often referred to as the "Big Five," this concept has been applied to the study of leadership. The Big Five are:

1. Openness—curious, original, and open to new ideas;
2. Conscientious—organized, systematic, punctual, achievement oriented, and dependable;
3. Extraversion—assertive, energetic, outgoing, talkative, and social;
4. Agreeableness—affable, tolerant, sensitive, trusting, kind, and warm;
5. Neuroticism—anxious, irritable, temperamental, and moody.

   T.A. Judge and his group have provided a comprehensive qualitative and quantitative review of this body of research [4]. His group found that extraversion, openness to experience, and conscientiousness positively correlated with leadership. Emerging as a leader was most strongly correlated with extraversion. Given the number of studies in his meta-analysis, one can reasonably conclude that these features play an important role in leadership.

Myers–Briggs

Another psychometric approach is to look at combinations of traits. Based on Jungian personality typologies, Myers–Briggs developed the "Type Indicator," a questionnaire that identifies what they call four ways of experiencing the world:

1. How you direct your energy, (I) introversion, preferring to deal with ideas and information, vs. (E) extroversion, preferring to deal with people, things, and the outer world;
2. How you process information, (S) sensing and dealing with facts vs. (N) intuition, dealing with ideas, possibilities, the unknown, and potential;
3. How you make decisions, (T) thinking and using objective logic, analytic, and detached vs. (F) feeling and using personal values and beliefs of what is important;
4. How you organize your life, (J) judging, planned, stable, and organized, vs. (P) perceiving, going with the flow, maintaining flexibility, and responding to things as they arise.

Each person is scored on each dimension and, if the four scores are combined, the test yields sixteen different personality types. Thus, an ENTJ would score highest on extraversion vs. introversion, intuition vs. sensing, thinking vs. feeling, and judging vs. perceiving.

The Myers–Briggs test is available online. Try taking it now. After taking the test, you can read about yourself and your way of experiencing the world. You can then probe further and find out what other world leaders or artists you resemble as well as gain insight into you weaknesses and strengths.

> As an aside, I took a leadership development course at one time with fourteen newly minted deans of U.S. medical schools. I found it astonishing that twelve of the fourteen of us tested as ENTJ. ENTJs have a natural tendency to "marshal and direct".... "I don't care to sit by the window on an airplane. If I can't control it, why look?" [5]

Judge's meta-analysis is so exhaustive and the Myers–Briggs so widely used that we can use their findings as a basis with which to assess how they play out in the context of the AMC, based on our experience. We will take up Judge's traits—extraversion, conscientiousness, and openness—and comment on their usefulness as well as potential pitfalls. With Myers–Briggs, we will comment on useful ways we have found to interpret and use the test.

Extraversion/Introversion and How It Plays Out in the AMC

The concept of extraversion is about energy and a propensity to seek interaction with people and the outside world, whereas introversion is about gaining energy in solitude or in the pursuit of ideas and information.

> I recall soon after becoming a chair that I was impressed with how much "pressing the flesh" was involved. I locked on to the image of a politician, working a crowd, and thought, "Man, don't do this if you don't like kissing babies."

Leadership in the AMC requires the ability to go out and meet with people in a variety of settings with a widely diverse set of interests and priorities. This is especially true as one moves up the administrative ladder. The requirements are greatest on the dean and less so with the chair or division head.

> As a dean, I would be out two nights a week and a weekend day most of the time. And this was after spending nearly all day every day in meetings. I'd be asked to speak to alumni groups, donors, legislators, supporters of the university (and a few critics), as well as recruits, faculty, university trustees and so forth. Nearly every archival photograph of a dean will show him or her at a reception talking to someone.

It also takes energy to get out and sell an idea. Moving people along to get buy-in for a new idea requires jawboning and talking through the same point again and again with different people. As a historical case in point, Martin Luther King, Jr., who is often credited with the leadership speech of the century with his "I Have a Dream" speech, subsequently gave that same speech 60 times in the following year.

Extraverts have the advantage here because they keep or even gain energy with human interactions, whereas introverts tire out. Introverts need to be alone to recover and re-energize. Leadership doesn't require complete extraversion, but there must be enough so that meeting with people doesn't wear you out.

It's not hard to find those with enough extraversion and those with too much introversion. Introverts will leave large groups early and come late just in time to give a preprogrammed speech. Meanwhile, the extravert will get there early and mix and mingle with the crowd and then use the information gleaned to include in his or her extemporaneous remarks. This contrast between Bill Clinton and Al Gore was a hallmark of their differences in personality styles and traits. Clinton may have been habitually late to show up for social events, but he had the reputation for being among the last to leave—Gore was the opposite. In fact it is said that the Secret Service sometimes had great difficulty protecting Gore because of his tendency to withdraw from events and seek isolation.

However, in our experience, we don't find introversion, in and of itself, to be disqualifying. In fact, it has some advantages in the right circumstance. The introvert is more comfortable in small groups and favors more formalized settings over informal ones. In a formalized setting, the introvert will be called on and, just as importantly, will know when he is being called on and for what purpose. In these circumstances he or she can dazzle with his or her organization and thoughtfulness.

Further, in a world of increasing uncertainty and ambiguity, where past experience can count for less, the ability to listen, absorb, process, and synthesize new information becomes paramount. These receptive–reflective skills are typically found more frequently with introverts.

Judge offers some pretty solid evidence that extraversion provides a natural advantage in leadership positions. But in the AMC where ideas are so valued that being introverted is not necessarily disabling, the question is whether you have enough extraversion. If you are comfortable in groups, if you can mingle and make extemporaneous remarks, if you can make small talk at sporting events, if you can chat with individuals or small groups, and if you hold up to a day full of meetings, at least two nights and a weekend day, then you have enough extraversion. If not, then you will need to compensate.

There are two ways an introvert can compensate. One, he or she can take this introversion into account in terms of how business is done, and second, he or she can add more extraverted people to the leadership team. Introverts do better if they have vice chiefs who can do the mixing and greeting and conversing. The introverted leader can then receive reports from an inner circle and determine a course of action. After considering all sides of an issue, the introvert does well to post all reports on the Internet so faculty can read them. This provides a sense of transparency that his or her personality doesn't naturally afford.

In fact, as a general rule, the smart money seems to be on encouraging diversity— partnerships and complementary styles can be very powerful, i.e., Honda/Fujisawa, Walt Disney/Roy Disney, and Don Keough/Roberto Goizueta are all classic examples. It can require balancing and delicate orchestration to pull this off, but it can be a critical variable during times of opportunity and crisis.

However, it may be possible to be too introverted for a leadership position, so the corresponding question is whether there can be too much extraversion. Certainly, if "too much" means impulsiveness or talking over people, then you have a problem.

This raises an important point. The issue of associated traits or characteristics is a great bugaboo in discussions of personality. Negative traits that are often associated with introversion are perfectionism, conflict aversion, and indecision; those associated with extraversion are impulsiveness and talking over people.

However, while certain traits may appear to cluster together, they are in fact independent of one another.

Thus, in this book, we will consider each characteristic on its own and not as part of the underlying extraversion or introversion. We take up conflict, impulsiveness, aversion, and indecision in Chap. 13, Making Good Decisions. Talking through or over people is considered in Chap. 6 on The Importance of Emotional Intelligence in the section on Validating While Listening.

In conclusion, extraversion and introversion continually appear in the literature as important variables in understanding leadership. We argue that you need enough extraversion but that compensatory strategies can be put in place to make up for a relative lack of extraversion. And, further, introversion has its own strengths and so should not be disqualifying on its own.

Thus, it's not so much whether you are extraverted or introverted or show any of the requisite traits that are hypothesized but rather whether you have enough of what is needed in the particular context of the organization and whether you can compensate for the rest. Ancona makes this point quite nicely in her article, "In Praise of the Incomplete Leader"; it is recommended for your reading [6].

Conscientiousness: Organized, Systematic, Punctual, Achievement Oriented, and Dependable, and How Conscientiousness Plays Out in the AMC

It's hard to argue with the importance of these characteristics to leadership. All make for a predictable work environment. If the boss says he or she is going to do something and doesn't, morale suffers. On the other hand, if you can count on him or her, a feeling of certainty is added to the environment. However, two characteristics require additional comment.

The first is punctuality. We've seen otherwise extraordinarily conscientious leaders of academic institutions being late for meetings rather regularly. They can be organized, conscientious, and achievement oriented but still be late consistently. They rarely see the negative effects. They will come to a meeting late that can't start without them and not be aware of how angry the group is. People feel disrespected when they are made to wait, and being late is experienced as an insult. The subtext message you are sending is that I am more important than you, and your time is less valuable than mine. It may not be what you think or say, but it's what others hear. Even if you are not essential for the group to start, when you are late, the group gets the obvious message that this meeting is not valued.

A second reason to be punctual is this. If you start a meeting on time regularly and if you end it on time regularly, people will come on time (well, most people will). If you start late regularly, people will come late. Operant conditioning does work, even with faculty.

We also need to comment about perfectionism. Perfectionism may be viewed as an extreme form of conscientiousness, or it can be viewed as a trait independent of conscientiousness. Regardless of how it is viewed, it can be a limiting personality trait. It is considered further later in these chapters on personality.

Openness: Curious, Original, and Open to New Ideas, and How Openness Plays Out in the AMC

Openness is a prerequisite to meeting the central tenets of this book. If authority is earned, it is only earned by being open to others' ideas. If you buy into the precept that the intellectual expertise resides in the lower levels of the organization, then openness to ideas is a necessity to confirm its legitimacy.

If knowledge of culture and the informal organization is essential to developing a winning strategy, then the ability to extract, that is, being open to, the values that form the culture and underlie behavior is essential.

While openness is obviously a central theme of this book, two unintended consequences should be considered. First, openness can lead to a dilution of purpose. Moving in too many new directions at one time will confuse the organization and can lead to defeat of initiatives. An organization can only move in a limited number of directions at once.

> I came to this by accident. We were having a clinic advisory meeting and our clinic director was outlining several initiatives that we had to accomplish as an organization. The discussion was going along with one cohort who were earnestly discussing the issues while a second contingent was being really picky about the details of what appeared to me to be reasonable and straightforward initiatives. The group began moving all over the map. Frustrated by the incoherence, I simply stated my priorities. "Look we have two priorities for the year: 1. Our finances, and 2. Patient satisfaction scores." I thought no more about it. Later in the year when we did our budget reviews, several commented on how helpful isolating just two objectives were. I was surprised at first but then it made sense. Don't confuse people with too many priorities.

Second, we've commented that as you ascend the administrative hierarchy, from division head to chair or to dean, you move further from your own area of expertise and become more dependent on others' ideas. But this openness can make you feel obsolete because you really are becoming obsolete from a technical perspective. But at the same time, you are becoming proficient in a series of skills, such as building teams, getting results, and pulling people together. While these skills are very real and separate good from average leaders, we don't have a ready way of talking about them. As a result, you may feel both a sense of obsolescence and an inability to describe what you can do, so you can easily feel and sound pretty lame and clichéd.

Myers–Briggs and How It Plays Out in the AMC

In our experience, the major benefit of the Myers–Briggs is that it provides the group a common vocabulary with which to talk about personality. Finding a way to get people to open up and talk about themselves and their personalities in a nondefensive way is essential to becoming a better leader. In fact, becoming comfortable with talking about yourself is more important than learning your specific personality profile, ENTJ, or whatever.

A second hoped-for outcome is that the leader sees that while people are different in how they process information, all the processes are valid. The Myers–Briggs can help people who are high on intuition (N) see how people who are high on sensing (S) might frustrate them with fact-filled, linear explanations. Or that (J)s' need for order and stability might get frustrated with (P)s' "go-with-the-flow" mentality. Learning that people who frustrate you are just different in how they process information and make decisions and are not inferior is an extremely valuable lesson.

In our classes, a third objective is to try getting participants to realize that their strongest points might become blind spots. Since our classes are often high in (N), it is important for them to see how their use of intuition might make them move too quickly, when a more extended visit with the facts (S) might be appropriate. Learning that strengths can become weaknesses is also an important lesson.

Review of biographical information and psychometric tests, we believe, leads to this: you can argue about whether traits are immutable and which traits are most important to a leader, though you'd be just a little ornery if you didn't factor in "enough" extraversion, conscientiousness, and openness. But even if you disregard these, the more important issue is whether you understand the traits you have and whether you can adapt them to circumstance and context. Can you compensate for your weaknesses, not become blinded by your preferred methods of processing information and making decisions, and find a way to enhance the contributions of others by deploying their strengths? If you can, you have the personality it takes to be a really good leader.

References

1. Erikson E. Young Man Luther. New York: Peter Smith Publishers; 1962. p. 124.
2. Psychometric Tests. 2015. http://www.psychometrictest.org.uk/big-five-personality/
3. The Myers & Briggs Foundation, Florida, 2015. http://www.myersbriggs.org/my-mbti-personality-type/mbti-basics/
4. Judge TA, Bono JE, Ilies R, Gerhardt MW. Personality and leadership: a qualitative and quantitative review. J Appl Psychol. 2002;87(4):765–80.
5. Humanmetrics. ENTJ Description. http://www.humanmetrics.com/personality/entj
6. Ancona D, Malone T, Orlikowski W, Senge P. In praise of the incomplete leader. Harv Bus Rev. 2007;85(2):92–100.

Chapter 5
Managing Personality Disorders in the Workplace

People with personality disorders wreak havoc in the workplace because they interfere with work, disrupt relationships, extract high levels of energy from co-workers and undermine the potential for maintaining a positive working environment. Leaders typically dread dealing with these dysfunctional sometimes toxic personalities. We know of no retired leader who isn't glad to leave these people to his or her successor.

Personality disorders differ from traits because they are more severe and have the capacity to interfere with success and happiness in life. We select three for consideration here because they seem to thrive in the AMC and because in our experience they are the ones that occur most frequently. They are narcissism, passive–aggressiveness, and perfectionism.

Narcissism

Leaders of AMCs would do well to understand narcissism and how to work with it—both their own and others' narcissism. In our experience coaching, this psychological concept resonates the most and is the most easily applied and understood.

Narcissus, according to Greek mythology, was a beautiful man. As the legend goes, he saw his reflection in a pool of water and fell in love with it. According to various versions, he finally died (or committed suicide) when he realized it was only an image and he could not have the object of his desire.

Accordingly, narcissism has come to refer to absorption with oneself and one's desires. As a personality disorder, it is characterized by grandiosity, the need for admiration, and a sense of entitlement [1]. It becomes a personality disorder when it interferes with effectiveness at work, or with interpersonal relationships.

However, all narcissism is not bad. There is the good (healthy) and then the bad (unhealthy) narcissism, which is expressed as a personality disorder.

© Springer International Publishing Switzerland 2015
J.L. Houpt et al., *Learning to Lead in the Academic Medical Center*,
DOI 10.1007/978-3-319-21260-9_5

Healthy narcissism, or stable positive self-esteem, is the stuff that gives you the self-confidence so important to leadership. It allows you to stand before a group and give a speech, to enter a legislator's office whom you don't know and argue your case, or to make a difficult decision that others might avoid. Adulation doesn't become an end in itself as it is with bad narcissism. The good narcissism can just be banked from the good days and used when needed. Without some healthy narcissism, no one would seek the position of a chair or dean.

When it occurs in the leader, the unhealthy narcissism manifests itself in a number of ways that limit his or her effectiveness. It leaves a number of distinctive footprints. Consider the dean (or chair or division head) who:

1. Can't be criticized (because the person has to be adored in every circumstance), thus cutting off any meaningful discussion;
2. Chooses weak members of his or her team because the sole criterion used is that the team support the leader's ego to make him or her feel powerful;
3. Removes the existing staff (they're not up to the leader's standards) and thus eliminates the institutional memory and goes on to make a string of decisions that violate the culture of the institution;
4. Cannot imagine any solution to a problem that doesn't glorify him or her, so that institutional priorities fall to the leader's personal ones;
5. Doesn't accept responsibility for making a mistake and so has to blame others;
6. Takes credit for all that is good and thus robs others of the recognition they deserve;
7. Takes a job just to pad a resume and actually has little interest in the institution or its faculty.

If the leader demonstrates any of these behaviors, the institution has to bend to him or her. The institution is virtually helpless to change the behaviors, short of the leader's flaws being discovered by his or her bosses. The reason why such a person is so infrequently ferreted out is that the narcissistic leader is a master of convincing his or her superiors that he or she is very special. Even if the leader is discovered and referred for coaching, the patterns are very hard to change. The relationship with the coach is complicated because the narcissist engages with the coach the way he or she engages with superiors—by presenting material aimed to impress the coach. Institutions can and do survive, but with diminished morale and effectiveness. It is far preferable that search committees screen these people out.

Narcissistic personalities live among the faculty as well as among the leaders of the AMC. They thrive within the academic milieu. Whether it's competing for grants or patients or membership in the most prestigious societies, or building the largest clinical program, or being invited to present in the most prestigious meeting, or being named to an endowed professorship, or a host of other things, there are daily reminders of one's standing and status. This type of culture can push healthy narcissism to the unhealthy side.

Within the faculty, narcissism expresses itself in wanting all resources for oneself, in anger and disappointment when one's boss doesn't "appreciate" him or her enough, and in narrow parochial thinking. It encourages people to think they are above the rules and don't need to put up with bureaucratic nitpickings, e.g., signing charts, or even the need to deal with "inferiors" civilly.

The goal is diminishing the effect that narcissists exert on the work environment. To do so, you need to understand a few things about them. First, narcissists are the way they are because they have to constantly support their (compensatory) inflated view of themselves. One such leader was described by his direct reports as "a self-made man, who worships his creator." While they may appear off the charts to you with regard to how pleased they are with themselves, they can only sustain it through creating an environment that reinforces it. A measure of their underlying insecurity is how an innocuous remark can enrage them because it means you haven't seen how important they really are. So think of these "big egos" as compensated "weak egos" with underlying insecurities and self-doubts.

Second, the behavior patterns that make up a personality disorder are invisible to the person with the personality disorder. For the most part, they think they are fine. They think you are the problem. For example, from your perspective, you might see someone as seriously entitled. But, from their perspective the problem is that you don't appreciate them enough. Only occasionally and only after repeated insults to their personal happiness or success do they even begin to feel anxiety or depression and begin to wonder if they are the problem. But usually they continue blithely along, blaming other people.

The third feature of this personality disorder follows from the first two. The behaviors of the person with a personality disorder don't bother him or her, but they irritate others. It's the other people who feel the pain and get frustrated. It's the other people who go home angry or lash out in response and embarrass themselves.

Your focus as a leader needs to be on mitigating the noxious effect of the narcissist on the work environment. You need to manage the narcissist. Since narcissists are the way they are in order to support their inflated view of themselves, the first goal of management requires supporting their self-esteem: "I really appreciate your point of view," "that was a great presentation today," "even though I need to rule against your idea, I still think it was great," "we're far better off by having you on our faculty," and "your ideas were right on point as always, however, in this case...."

The best medicine is to treat everyone as if they are narcissists, whether they are or not. Erring on the side of positive feedback has some definite advantages.

> It took me far too long to figure out the simple idea that if you didn't tell them it was good, they'll never know you thought it was good. I also learned over time that positive feedback shapes behavior more powerfully than negative feedback. If you make clear expectations and give positive feedback, not just that person, but also others will go that direction. If your method of setting expectations is criticism, people will only fight you.
>
> There may be a number of reasons why people don't compliment people enough. Some were raised where you were expected to do things the right way, so no comments were needed unless you did things wrong. It may also be a function of the fact that it is really hard in complex political organizations to give people honest compliments or positive feedback without appearing to be a sycophant. Thus people avoid it, and as a result a lot of people I think are starved for that occasional confirmation or praise that we all need.

The second goal of management is to avoid massive and severe confrontation. What you never want to do is to break through someone's defenses with some cutting criticism and land a blow to the person's self-esteem (even though that's what you want to do when he or she has angered you). If you display anger, you unleash a torrent of rage in response from them, which you will never be able to undo. Their anger is called "narcissistic rage." It can be very severe.

> I have unfortunately unleashed it at times, and I can best describe it as saying I can feel the hate they have for me viscerally. If you ever wonder what you have done to that person so that they hate you so much, the likely answer is that you inflicted a narcissistic injury and unleashed their rage.

The third strategy is to not get drawn into the drama. Remember, narcissistic people feel no pain; they want you to feel it. Said simply, don't let these people get under your skin. Your own response of annoyance, frustration, or anger can only hurt you. If it occurs in a group setting, you are seen as not in control emotionally. Even if it occurs alone in a private setting, they know that they got to you and can control you.

The fourth strategy is to only get involved when the narcissist is interfering with the work of the group. If this happens, your only focus should be getting the work done. Whether people have personality disorders or not is not your problem. That's the province of a psychotherapist. Your only concern should be getting the work of the group done.

Let us illustrate this with a case example. Let's assume you are leading a group meeting where the "work" of the group is to plan a genomics program. The immediate subject is financing, and it becomes obvious that funding genomics will inevitably curtail any new money for other programs for some time. Now, as a hypothetical, recall the faculty member mentioned earlier who screamed at the business manager that "any money not going to me is wasted." Imagine that the faculty member is objecting to such a program because "we are doing so well and have so many excellent programs going that I don't think that putting the money into genomics now is a good idea. Let's just continue as we are and wait on this."

Whether it's in a group setting or in a private meeting, the initial response is the same. First, don't get flustered and don't blurt out "you self-centered egomaniac" even though you might be thinking it. You might simply respond, "Our strategic plan determined that our most important priority for NOW is genomics, and that's what we all agreed to do. That doesn't mean we can't do something else another time." If that works, say no more.

If you are in a group setting and the person comes back with some rejoinder, then he or she has raised the ante and is challenging your authority as group leader. Again the response is the same, don't let him or her see you sweat, and find a way to reiterate your point. Say, for example, "you are acting like this is the first discussion of this. This has been thoroughly reviewed by three faculty groups and voted on. We can't accomplish anything if we are going to go back and reverse the work of three different faculty reviews based on one person's unhappiness."

It's important to understand what this intervention has accomplished. You kept your cool and you have stated nothing but what is obvious to the whole group. But what you have done is making the person a deviant not just from you but also from the group. Further, you played the "emotional card" of the individual's not respecting his or her fellow group members and their opinions. This should keep the group on your side, which was what his play was all about anyway—to get the group against you.

Passive–Aggressive Personality

The second personality disorder we should consider is the passive–aggressive personality. Passive–aggressive people abound in the AMC. Though it is no longer a DSM-V category, understanding it continues to be useful in the AMC. In a word, these people just don't support or carry out the game plan. Often they don't take you on directly. They sit in meetings and say nothing. After a vote is taken, they leave the room quietly, but they just don't do whatever was decided to do. When it becomes obvious that after several trials they are not doing it, they may then tell you why it's not possible and have 80 reasons why it's someone else's fault.

They abound in AMCs because the cultures allow it. As we have said in Chap. 1, when you are in an environment where authority is distributed, and it is nearly impossible to ensure accountability, these people thrive. They can resist and resist forever, and there is always someone else to blame when things don't happen. They also thrive in environments where there is an attempt to maintain civility and avoid conflict. In these environments where public disagreement is frowned on, the most effective way to obstruct is to do so passively as a snake in the grass. If the leader is particularly conflict adverse, this is an added incentive for the passive–aggressive person to oppose whatever he or she doesn't agree with.

The approach here is in keeping with what we said earlier about people with personality disorders not feeling the pain even though you do. The first line of response is to not let them get under your skin. Control whatever anger you might feel. Aside from that, giving time lines with objective endpoints may help. You might also employ the strategy of getting everyone in the room when you set the time lines so that their responsibility is publicly known.

Once their resistance to the direction is clear to all, you can ask these individuals to get with the program or replace them with people who will do the job. After enough iteration, their passive resistance is brought out into the light for all to see.

Perfectionistic Personality

Conscientiousness is a valued trait, but perfectionism is not. There are two areas of difficulty for perfectionists: (1) they don't delegate well and instead micromanage and (2) they give too much negative feedback.

With regard to delegating, the perfectionist thinks, "I might as well do it myself because it's just easier than waiting for them to figure it out and then I have to correct them." That strategy may have worked for them when they were in smaller jobs, like their clinical practice or running their lab, but doesn't work when running a larger more complex unit like a department or the school.

In addition to just not working in larger groups, those who live with the motto that "it's just easier for me to do it" rob the group of any feeling of worthiness. If that attitude takes over, and the leader shies away from any faculty or staff input, the leader will demoralize and then antagonize the entire group. Think of this as a narcissistic injury inflicted on a group, unleashing group rage.

Trusting only himself or herself, the perfectionist works harder and longer alone and then puts the "perfect" product before the faculty, only to have them reject it because the individual "got no input from any of us" and "doesn't respect our opinion." Over multiple repeats of this process, the faculty detests the "arrogance" of the leader/perfectionist.

The poor delegator's problem is that he or she sees only the product as important, not the importance of process and buy-in. When thrust into a leadership position, this type doesn't see that the position involves motivating the group to do a good job. A leader like this still thinks it's the product itself, and so he or she takes it over. In addition to robbing the group of initiative, these are the people who become burnt-out micromanagers.

The second problem with perfectionists is that they give too much negative feedback. Since no job is done as well as they could, they give ongoing criticism to get the "perfect" product. As a result, they are constantly correcting people, which has the effect of draining all the energy from them and leads to resentment toward the perfectionist. The common refrain is, "every time I see him or her, I think I am being judged and that I'm coming up short."

Another problem with perfectionists is that they tend to view people as perfect or not. They don't see that all people have strengths and weaknesses and that skilled leadership places people in situations where they can succeed. By placing people in situations that match their skills, you can shape their behavior by complimenting them on what they've done well. Remember the adage that "a compliment is like a kiss through a veil." Learn to do it. It's amazing how hard people will work for you if you compliment and praise them and how little they will do if you constantly criticize them.

If you are a perfectionist, I'd suggest the following recipe: four tablespoons of praise for each tablespoon of criticism. In other words, if you are a perfectionist, you are allowed one criticism only after four compliments.

Before we end this section, I need to repeat a point made earlier. As a psychiatrist, who was a dean, I can recount numerous times when a problem was described to me as due to a personality disordered person when it wasn't. Labeling a person as having a personality disorder was being used as a way to discredit people, and absolve the describer/accuser of any responsibility. It's a way of blaming someone else. Thus your antenna should immediately go up when you are told that someone's view shouldn't be heard because they are "personality disordered". You should wonder if there isn't some truth to their objections and try to understand what is behind their views. Maybe you are missing something. As in the case of the chair in Chap. 2, the action of the dean was the same – to enact the cuts – but the approach differed when she understood the reasons behind his objections. Further, by understanding his reasons, she understood what the resistance from other chairs would be. Much would have been lost if she had just accepted that he was "passive-aggressive".

Reference

1. American Psychiatric Association. Diagnostic and statistical manual of mental disorders. 4th ed. 2000 June.

Chapter 6
The Importance of Emotional Intelligence

The concept of multiple intelligences dates to Howard Gardner and his 1983 book, *Frames of Mind* [1]. In it, he argues against there being just one kind of intelligence and against the traditional test of IQ as a monolithic measure of intelligence. Instead he proposes at least seven varieties of intelligence: 1. verbal, 2. mathematical (both comprising the traditional IQ test), 3. spatial capacity (the kind of intelligence demonstrated by an architect or artist), 4. kinesthetic (sports star or dancer), 5. musical (Beethoven), 6. interpersonal (knowledge of what goes on between people), and 7. intrapersonal (what goes on within a person).

These latter two—interpersonal and intrapersonal—comprise emotional intelligence (EI). It was popularized by Daniel Goleman with a spate of books for the business world arguing that certain interpersonal and intrapersonal skills accounted for the relative success or failure of business leaders [2]. Goleman breaks EI down into five areas: self-awareness, self-regulation, motivation, empathy, and social skills (p. 318). They provide the substrate from which one can learn a set of emotional competencies (EC) that provides the skills for success (pp. 26–27). We recommend his work to you.

In Goleman's lexicon:

Self-awareness (EI) makes possible the ability to assess one's strengths and weaknesses;
Self-regulation (EI) is necessary for self-control and adaptability;
Motivation-drive (EI) is the basis for initiative;
Empathy (EI) allows for political awareness, understanding others, and service orientation; and
Social skills (EI) are necessary for persuasion, communication, and inspiring others.

We have selected three emotional competencies based on our experience. They are (1) listening and (2) other-centeredness, both based on empathy, and (3) demeanor, based on self-regulation.

© Springer International Publishing Switzerland 2015
J.L. Houpt et al., *Learning to Lead in the Academic Medical Center*,
DOI 10.1007/978-3-319-21260-9_6

Validating While Listening

There are two aspects to this EI. One is listening; the second is validating the person's point of view. Listening while validating is largely dependent on the EI of empathy, probably formed early in life. Empathy is the ability to feel as other people feel. It is not feeling sorry for people's misfortune or showing sympathy. People may express sympathy because it is socially called for but not be able to feel another's pain. Psychopaths lack empathy, but they can be charming and be quite capable of expressing sympathy if it's in their best interest. Empathy involves an understanding of where the person is emotionally. And it is that capacity that permits one to formulate a response that is validating to another.

Listening requires that other people know that you have heard what they said. They won't know whether you hear unless you tell them that you did. Good leaders have to communicate in a way that demonstrates that they understand the content and appreciate the value of the points of view of the group.

> People's response to the idea that they need to listen better is amusing. When I'm at a reception and people ask me what I do, I tell them, "leadership development and coaching". A frequent response is, with some derision, "oh, you tell people to listen better". When I have a new client and I've just completed a 360, and I inform the client that people think they need to listen better, they often argue and say it's not true. Even when I tell them that this is why people hired me to help them, they deny it as a possibility.

Given people's reluctance to view themselves as poor listeners, the first step for new leaders is to ascertain whether they are good listeners. Actually, this is easy. The only way to know if you're a good listener is if others say you are. If they say you're not, you're not. As usual, perception is reality in the leadership context.

In a surprising number of cases, the profile of poor listeners is almost identical. They are almost always described as "bright" and "very intelligent." They make decisions quickly, they're excellent debaters, and they argue to win, not to understand. It's their rapidity of retort that earns them the descriptor "very intelligent," and it is often the reason why they win debates. Many mortals can't keep up with the speed. To make it worse, they often create a sense that they find you inferior after they have whipped you in a debate.

In addition, poor listeners share the same misperception. They think the purpose of a discussion is for *them* to come to a decision, not for *us* to come to a decision. They lose interest in the conversation when they have enough information to make their decision. This combination of thinking that they listen only to get information to make a decision and their natural proclivity to process information rapidly leads to off-putting behavior. They start talking over you and finishing your sentences, or they display an irritation with your slowness, and the discussion is over.

Poor listeners miss the fact that conversations have as a goal not only determining the right course of action but also simultaneously getting buy-in from others. That can only occur when others feel that their ideas and anxieties have been spoken to. Poor listeners just don't get that the secondary purpose of listening, and the one most crucial to bonding and building alliances, is to validate other people-to let them know not just that their words have been heard but that the importance they attach to the words has been received as well. People who leave a room feeling that you respect them and their ideas feel like they have been heard, even if you disagree with their ideas. People want to be respected. Faculty in academia have chosen a life where their thoughts are paramount to their success and thus to their self-esteem. Poor listeners, by showing little respect for others' ideas, actually assault others' self-esteem. And faculty then respond with anger toward such poor listeners.

Excellent listeners differ from poor listeners in other ways as well. Really good listeners can suspend final judgment while they hear other views. All of you strong Js on the Myers–Briggs pay attention to this: good listeners mentally try out the fit of others' views against their own. To them, an idea is always open to modification. It's not that they don't have ideas; they do, but an idea can always be enriched.

Good listeners have a basic respect for all people and all opinions. They see people not as smart or dumb or right or wrong but as coming from different places, which is a lesson to learn from Myers–Briggs. They place opinions within a context rather than in absolute terms. Poor listeners look to see whether others agree or disagree with them and then conclude that they are smart or dumb.

It also helps to be able to listen to criticism nondefensively and to be willing to tolerate conflict. If you add an aversion to conflict and an inability to tolerate the expression of negative feelings to a lack of respect for people, you have a deadly combination.

> Some people are good listeners; others are less so. I doubt the poor listeners can ever be brought up to the level of the good listeners, but all of us can become better listeners if we work on it.
>
> For some, their "original" empathy has been lost. Medical education can socialize individuals in the wrong directions. Over the years they've gotten in a hurry and can't waste time with non-productive conversations, have gotten enamored of their intelligence and speed, and have gotten away with bullying people with it. In my experience, they require a large amount of confrontation to accept the need to change. However, with enough confrontation, and with making convincing arguments that they could be even more effective if they make some changes, they can improve.
>
> They need also to change their assumption of what a conversation is about. The purpose of the conversation includes bringing other people along with a decision. If you enter the discussion having already a pretty firm idea of your decision, you should listen to see if you could improve or refine your decision. At the least, you need to affirm the value of others' views so that when they leave the room, they say, "he or she got it". This is a critical part of implementing any new initiative. Without this validation there is no buy-in, and there is very little chance that the leader's ideas can be implemented.
>
> You need to adopt a strategy to end every interview with an action plan. Summarize what you heard and ask the other person if you missed anything. State what the next step is, that is, "I'll need to consult with some people and I'll have so and so get back to you", or "let me know if anything new arises". The point is that an action plan confirms that you have heard what they have said. If you don't have any idea what to do, just say "thank you for bringing this to my attention; let me think on it."

Other-Centeredness: It's Not About You, and the Search for People Who Experience Pleasure in Others' Doing Well

Other-centeredness is another quality based on the EI of empathy, just as listening is. James Collins, in his book, *Good to Great* [3], studied 28 companies to ascertain why some leveled out at "good," while others went on to be "great." He found a number of differences, but a major factor was the "level 5 leader." The companies that jumped from being good to being great had a level 5 leader. Level 5 leaders channel their ego needs away from themselves and into the larger goal of building a great company. It's not that level 5 leaders have no ego or self-interest. Indeed, they are incredibly ambitious—but their ambition is first and foremost for the institution, not themselves (p. 21).

Collins goes on to say that great leaders don't talk about themselves. They attribute success to others within the organization, but take the blame when things go wrong.

On the other side of the spectrum, there is the self-centered leader. Collins calls these people I-centric. To Collins they are the opposite of the level 5 leader: self-aggrandizing, taking credit for whatever good happens and shifting blame to others when things go wrong, lacking humility, and always building their resume. You will recognize these traits as part of what we described as unhealthy narcissism.

Other-centeredness is not the same as altruism to our thinking. The altruist is one who does well for no personal benefit. It requires a near-perfect state of selflessness. These people are in short supply in the AMC, so don't count on them. What we want are people who feel excitement when others get a grant, make a clinical breakthrough, and get an award or when a student finally gets it. These people are not selfless. They are energized and full of themselves when others do well. We should be looking for people who experience pleasure when others do well, even when they surpass us.

Theorists disagree as to how and when someone acquires the capacity to put the interests of others ahead of his or her own. One view is that it's developmental. Erikson proposed that we age into it [4]. He thought that about the age of 40, one entered a period of life where one is thrust between the two poles of generativity and stagnation. It is a period of life well known to those in the AMC. Is my research going okay or is it slipping? Should I continue on or change course? Can I keep my lab alive? Can I keep up the clinical pace? Should I extend a lab or clinical practice by bringing others in and increasing my sphere of influence by mentoring my colleagues and developing them? This tension between generativity and stagnation can be a powerful impulse toward moving to a position of taking pleasure in others. It requires a shift of locus of the source of satisfaction and gratification from yourself to others. It needs be no less gratifying than doing it all yourself. A second point of view is that other-centeredness is evident as early as 3 or 4 years of age. There are kids who share their toys and work to include all kids in play so that everyone has a good time. They know everyone's favorite color and food preference. Meanwhile, other kids hoard their toys and have no clue what anyone else's preferences are. They are either other focused or I-focused that early.

Whenever and however it develops, the surest way to ensure the success of your AMC is to recruit level 5 leaders. It is much easier to recruit them than to try to add to a behavioral repertoire that was lacking in a person already hired in a leadership position.

However, there is another aspect to this concept of other-centeredness. It focuses not just on the interests of the individual but also on the group. The issue is whether the people within the institution can put the institution ahead of their own self-interest and whether the groups within the institution, say a department, can deny their interests for the good of the larger institution.

Moving Beyond Self-Interest and Creating an Interest in the Larger Institution

> I believe that institutions take on some of the characteristics of the leader. If you care for others and if you have the institution at heart, you have at least earned the right to ask the group to move in certain directions with you. If you wish to be a transformational leader, you need to be able to do this.

This other-centeredness is not a natural resting point when you consider the nature of individuals and groups. By their nature, individuals and groups are centered on their self-interests. You will recall that the first job of the leader is to help the group survive and prosper. You will recall also that academic institutions have demanded independence above all else in determining promotion and tenure. As a result, the natural flow is first toward individuals and their careers and then second to their immediate group, e.g., division or department. The third consideration is the institution.

What separates leaders from managers is the ability to take the group from its smallish self-interest to a concern for the larger institution. It involves moving the group to a point that is not natural and requires a new commitment. It's really hard for leaders to do that if they, too, are self-interested. The group needs to see that its leader is interested in the larger group and the institution. It's much easier to say, "Join me," than to say, "Don't do what I do, do what I say." As a group bonds to a leader, they will take on his or her characteristics.

There are also other things that can be done to move the group from its smallish self-interest to a grander and broader view.

First, don't be dispirited when you see people seeking their own self-interest or their department's self-interest. Appreciate that fighting for their unit is what the unit is demanding of the leader. But counter it calmly by pointing out that this issue is about the welfare of the institution. You must continually emphasize that point.

Second, take advantage of every opportunity to show the interdependence of the different units. Mention in your informal gatherings and in your faculty meetings the grants or clinical programs that involve more than one unit. If one unit makes a contribution to another or makes a sacrifice, then comment on it. In the clinical area, emphasize the downstream economics, e.g., primary care feeds orthopedics, which feeds radiology, which feeds the hospital.

Third, set up systems that explicitly reward teamwork.

Early in my career as a dean, I was asked by a chair candidate how I judged the chairs. My response was that you can make a B plus if you recruit well, support teaching, maintain morale, and balance the books. But if you want to make an A, you have to make the institution better.

That comment occurred in the early 1990's and was appropriate for that time. The model was strong chairs, growth, and superb recruitment. The thought was that everything would take care of itself if these things occurred. However, with the advent of managed care in the 90's, the changing methods of healthcare financing, and the emerging importance or interdisciplinary research, that model proved ineffective over the next decade.

What was called for was an integrated approach to healthcare and research, e.g. genomics, nanotechnology, spreading across departments and even schools. As a result, when asked by chair candidates a decade later what I expected from chairs, my answer was that they had to do two things: they had to take care of their department, recruit, support teaching, maintain morale, and balance the books, and second, they had to do so within the overall interests of the institution and in a way that supported the other departments. You need to be explicit about this, and you need to consider it in reviews of performance and compensation.

I consider the conflict between the individual's and the department's self-interest and the interests of the institution THE consuming problem in the current environment. One sees it repeatedly when the demands of the health system completely distort the normal architecture of the medical school and disturb the balance of patient care, research, and teaching. I see it on the research side when a field emerges, say genomics, that requires a huge shift of resources in that direction and away from existing departmental interests. And I see it in teaching when CMS releases guidelines for teachers that require an enormous increase in charting. Or when new IT systems are introduced and require six-month adaptations, with loss of revenue as a real potential.

All those examples require putting the institution first. This is what modern leadership is all about. You are fortunate if you have a cadre of other centered leaders, departmental and institutional, who can lead others to that point.

Self-Awareness/Demeanor and Consistent Style

William Osler, the noted physician, claimed that the most important element in being a great clinician was equanimity ("Aequanimitas") [5]. Just as patients need to feel that their physician is in control, so do all the constituents of the AMC with respect to their leader.

I was sitting on the dais outside the new Public Health building during its dedication. When I returned to my office I had an e-mail from a faculty member, saying, "You looked so depressed today at the dedication – are you okay?" I was astounded. In fact I was not depressed but I was preoccupied as I felt like I had so much work to do and here I was trapped for one hour on a stage where I had no function but to be there. This email made me aware of how important demeanor is. I've become convinced those faculties who like you fear that the job will be too much for you – maybe unconsciously that it will kill you. You need to reassure them otherwise by your demeanor.

I've noted on other occasions, such as receptions and the like, that the first words out of people's mouths that you haven't seen in a while are, "you look great – it looks like the job agrees with you." Or another time, "you look so relaxed".

I once toured the JFK Presidential Library in Quincy, Mass. In it there are a number of videos of the debate between JFK and Richard Nixon. In them, Nixon has a five o'clock shadow and looks tired and even worn out. JFK looks vigorous and in fine spirits. Interestingly people who saw the debate on TV thought that Kennedy won, whereas those that heard it on the radio thought the Nixon had won. So the issue of demeanor and how you look is important.

Part of a leader's demeanor is based on the EI of self-regulation. But, equanimity does not mean controlling all feelings. I've heard some people describing their leader as "lacking human juices". They are so controlled in their emotions that others don't feel any affinity for them.

Humor is a great indicator of having feelings, but also being in control of them. Some people can use humor effectively and others not. Observe groups collected in the hallway or lunchroom. In some there is a somber tone, whereas in others there is constant laughing and joking going on. But ineffective attempts at humor can be laden with aggression. They may also consist of banter, often incessant, that precludes ever getting to the issues.

But effective humor is benign relative to aggression and lifts and lightens what would other be a gruesome discussion. Further, if people can laugh at themselves, they can accept criticisms and learn from situations. I've tried to make it a rule in recruiting people to go out and have dinner and make sure that they can laugh. I tried not to hire humorless people.

Interestingly there is research that substantiates the importance of humor in leadership—it describes the positive correlation between executive humor, enhanced organizational performance, and higher bonuses for the executive with a sense of humor [6].

Some people lack presence. Perhaps it's not fair but they just aren't taken seriously. Groups want their leader to appear "Presidential." Some people bridle at the bit when they rise to a leadership position. They complain that they just want to be themselves. They see taking on a "Presidential" air as phony. Unfortunately for them, that is not what their constituencies want. Leaders need to accept that one responsibility of the job is appearing to be capable of doing the job.

Being "Presidential" is not the same as being distant or unapproachable. Far from it. As we've said earlier, earning authority requires a person who can comfortably relate to all constituencies. In everyday parlance what we are looking for are people who are comfortable in their own skin.

Having a relaxed and stable emotional baseline is important because deviations from it are often warning signals of too much stress. Becoming irritable, short-tempered, drinking too much, and not sleeping are all signs that you are heading into a danger zone. You need to recognize that early signs and find a way to recalibrate; take time off or delegate some issues from your plate so that is more manageable. You should know your earliest warning signs. I'm a big sleeper so when my sleep was disturbed I knew I had to move into action to clear my plate or delegate it to someone.

Like all of the three emotional intelligences we've covered, demeanor is to some degree hardwired. However, experience and an increased level of confidence permit some people to improve what they project.

We've taken a position in regard to the role of personality and emotional intelligence that acknowledges that they can limit effectiveness—in extreme cases they can be disqualifying—but in milder cases they are capable of being remedied with appropriate coaching or just plain learning on the job. People can get better at this. Life experiences can improve empathy and self-regulation, and compensatory mechanisms can be brought to bear on traits like introversion and many others that might be limiting. No one is perfect. All can get better.

References

1. Gardner H. Frames of mind: the theory of multiple intelligences. 3rd ed. New York: Basic Books; 2011.
2. Goleman D. Working with emotional intelligence. New York: Bantam Books; 1998.
3. Collins J. Good to great. New York: HarperCollins; 2001.
4. Erikson E. Childhood and society. W.W. Norton and Co. 1950; republished as a Penguin Book, 1969.
5. Osler W. Aequanimitas. Forgotten Books; 2012.
6. Boyatzis R, McKee A. Resonant leadership. Boston: HBR Press; 2006. p. 87–8.

Part III
Essential Skills

The first two parts have suggested that if you can learn to use the formal and informal organization, understand the culture, establish your authority, and not be disqualified by personality features or shortcomings in emotional intelligence, you can enhance your effectiveness as a leader. If you add to that some basic management skills: getting started, negotiating, recruiting, conflict resolution, persuasion, running a meeting, making good decisions, and stimulating change, you can learn to become even a better leader. Even if you can't master all the intricacies of culture, and even if your personality limitations are significant, you can still benefit by learning these management skills. Further, you will also become a more relaxed and confident leader.

Chapter 7
Getting Started the Right Way

The All Important First Year

The first year is the most important period in your tenure in a leadership position. The perceptions you generate and the decisions made about you in the first year are very hard to change. Bad first years often cannot be overcome. Even when they are, your overall effectiveness will be diminished.

If you successfully navigate this year, you will have accomplished the following:

- Earned your authority;
- Identified cultural beliefs and assumptions that will need to be worked with;
- Demonstrated many of the values that will define your time in office;
- Defined either the beginnings of a strategic plan or be even further along with a nearly complete plan for years 1 and 2;
- Come to understand the informal as well as formal organization;
- Put together a leadership team that has both policy and also implementation capacity.

You can enhance your chance of success by recalling that the role of the leader is first and foremost to convince the group that he or she can help them survive and thrive, that authority is earned, and that beliefs, values, and assumptions are very important. Your ability to apply those concepts can help with a successful first year and be a springboard to a successful longer term.

This chapter illustrates these concepts by focusing on three different but inter-locking areas: (1) avoiding rookie mistakes, (2) listening and learning, and (3) using the stump speech to build buy-in.

© Springer International Publishing Switzerland 2015
J.L. Houpt et al., *Learning to Lead in the Academic Medical Center*,
DOI 10.1007/978-3-319-21260-9_7

Avoiding Rookie Mistakes

The cardinal rookie mistake is to misread the culture. New leaders often act as if
they have a chip embedded in their limbic lobes that fires all the same behaviors that
worked in their previous place or position. They don't stop to ask whether they will
violate the norms in the new place/position. For example, here are three responses
to a new environment that are sure to antagonize.

**Rookie mistake #1: "At (fill in some previous prestigious place),
we did things this way…."**
In nearly every statement, you mention where you're from and how things were
done there. Such a statement implies that this is the way you'll be having them done
here. It further implies that your new colleagues don't know how to do things and
that you don't have much to learn from them. While that may not be what you
intend, this behavior is interpreted as disrespect and arrogance.

**Rookie mistake #2: "I've (or the president and I have) decided
that we need to…."**
Because you and the president agree on your "charge," and because you've met with
the search committee and know their views and that you were their choice, you as a
novice dean believe that you have a mandate. You announce it the first day and start
moving pieces to accomplish it. Whatever the president's charge is-increase NIH
funding, join the "top 10," develop a biotech center, gain market share in cardiology,
meet the manpower void for primary care physicians in rural areas, or whatever—
you are *not* ready to announce it as a strategic plan and start. To do so is naive. You
do not have buy-in from the faculty. They do not take orders. To use the military
metaphor, the faculty have to volunteer for service, and they will only do that after
they have accepted the new direction as their idea. Premature announcement of a plan
short-circuits the emotional attachment that is necessary for authority to be bestowed
on you. The lead-in paragraphs in Chap. 3 on Authority deal with this point.

  The same thing is true for a chair that moves prematurely on a plan that he or she
and dean concoct, or a division head with a plan that he or she and the chair concoct.
Faculty consultation and involvement in hatching the plan is always required.

Rookie mistake #3. "Your baby is ugly"
One of the hardest messages to give to a group is that they are deficient and need to
change. They hear it as "your baby is ugly." Good leadership often requires the ability to do this, but if at all possible deliver this message only after authority has been
bestowed on you. There may be circumstances where you have to begin this way,
like disasters requiring a quick turnaround, but most jobs don't start out in crisis
mode. These messages are hard in any circumstance, but they go down best after
you are established, after they know you care about them and respect them and after
they've been convinced that you have their best interests at heart.

  All three of these "mistakes" have a common theme. In all, you appear to be
disrespecting your new colleagues. Perceived disrespect cannot be emphasized
enough. Even if you don't intend it, and even if you don't feel it, appearing to

disrespect people is the cardinal sin in an academic setting. We value our intellect and ideas above all else, and our self-esteem depends on them. Any inkling that you disrespect your new colleagues will not only alienate them but also create enough anger to mobilize them to overthrow you.

> For all the many and complicated reasons that someone gets fired, in my experience as a coach, there is always an element of perceived disrespect. Even if it doesn't lead to being fired, it will thwart all your efforts, because you will not be embraced emotionally. People will not bond with you, and thus they will never take the hill when you issue the order to charge. They will never fight against those who might want to fire you.
>
> I learned about this from my wife. I was sitting at the breakfast table one day and began reviewing my schedule. I commented to her that I had to see so and so that day, and that I dreaded it because he hated me so intensely. I went on about how good I had been to this person, how I had gone out of my way to help, and how I didn't know why he still hated me. She looked up from her paper and asked, "what do you think of him?" I quickly blurted out that I thought "he was an idiot." "Duh" was her retort. I then went on to say how cleverly I had disguised this, when she interrupted me with "people know when you don't respect them."
>
> Since that time, I've watched this happen over and over again. People really do know when you don't respect them.

Rookie mistake #4. Looking after #1.
When your first move is seen as taking care of yourself—whether in the salary and perks you negotiate for yourself, or in lavish redecoration of your office, or in building a huge office staff before you have consulted the faculty and gotten buy-in for what you are going to do for them—you've made a major mistake. In fact, if you are going to have to engage in any cost cutting, to spend funds on your office or any other tangible trapping of office is highly risky.

You are bestowed the authority necessary to lead only if you convince the faculty that you have their best interests at heart. Focusing on yourself first, before doing something for the faculty, only signals that you view yourself, and not them, as #1.

Listen and Learn

The first task of a new leader is to listen and learn. You should take advantage of as many sources of information and advice as are available—meetings with all constituents, individually or in groups, faculty committees, external consultants, and perhaps with a coach you hire for yourself. The knowledge you seek is not just specifics of a plan—goals, objectives, the implementation plan, or the business plan. You want to know about all the factors covered in section one of this book—the informal and formal organizations, beliefs, assumptions, values, the varied constituencies (the microclimates), what motivates people, and more. None of this can you know when you walk into your job on day one.

The first year provides an ideal time to learn all of this because people expect it of you. They don't expect you to know everything at the beginning. If you miss this first year window, and try to do it later in your term, people will question what you are really up to, because they believe you should have mastered this knowledge by now.

However, even more important, the process of collecting information is not just about bits of information; it's about a powerful emotional process in which all constituents are deciding whether to trust you or not and whether they're willing to entrust themselves and the school to you. This emotional bonding is crucial to their willingness to follow you. You're not the leader if no one follows you. And ultimately that's what the first year is really about.

Meet and Greet

Because the first year should involve both information collection as well as emotional bonding, the most important meetings are face-to-face meetings. Whether a dean, chair, or division head, your primary focus should be the faculty, but other chairs/deans, alumni, donors, and village elders are also important.

> There are two approaches I've found useful in meeting and greeting. The first is a series of questions that work particularly well in one on one meetings or at the end of a group meeting where you want to move from generalizations to concrete proposals. The questions are fundamentally these: 1. where do you think I should be trying to take this institution, and 2. what do you think I should be focused on? Both of these are open-ended and permit the responder to go wherever he or she pleases. Much can be learned by just considering this information. Does everyone locate the problem in the clinical systems, or in the research program? Do significant numbers all identify the same problem, or are the responses all over the board?
>
> After these open-ended questions, you might then try to narrow the focus with these follow up questions: 1. what do you think is the single most important issue, or 2. specifically, what would I need to do for you to think I'd done a good job, and 3. would any of these things you've said be really hard or "third rail" issues?
>
> I must admit that I had no such clarity of purpose when I was dean or chair, but I have applied this set of questions in a number of settings as a coach for deans or chairs, and I have found it very valuable. I've been able to identify stakeholders who are only interested in their own department or fiefdom, and I've been able to tap the culture and identify low hanging fruit and third rail issues.
>
> You'd be amazed at the similarity of opinion. If for whatever reason you are not able to elicit this information (maybe because you are the boss and they're intimidated or fear reprisal), then hire a third person to get this information for you. It's out there, easy to acquire, and extraordinarily valuable.

The Stump Speech: From Stump Speech to Strategic Plan

You must have a stump speech. It serves several purposes. It acts as a starter to get discussions going, especially with groups of people. The stump speech also offers you an opportunity to show that you are aligned with them and to affirm their values. And finally, it also provides a vehicle for you to try out your ideas and get feedback before going public with your strategic plan.

Since so many of your meetings are in groups, and your goal in all these meetings is to get the constituents to talk, you need an opening statement. People want to know your thoughts. You need to say something about your vision, but you don't want it to sound like a conclusion—the end of the story. Instead, you need something that tells them where you are in your thinking but that keeps the door open.

Here are some hypothetical stump speeches.

A dean (outside selection): *I'm delighted to be your dean. I know I have a lot to learn about this place, but I want you to know that I've always respected it. I particularly have admired your commitment to excellence. But the quest for excellence implies that we're not happy where we are—we're going to build on what we have. We'll take a look at all our missions—teaching, research, and clinical enterprise— and we'll decide where we want to go. You'll be part of those decisions.*

A chair (outside selection): *I'm delighted to be your chair. I'm especially familiar with your division of cardiology since I have followed their work closely in that I've had to compete with them for grants. I'm happy we are now on the same team. I look forward to getting to know all the other divisions as well. We'll take a look at all of our missions and I'll depend on your advice as we move forward.*

A division head (inside selection): *We've known each other a long time and I just want to say that I'm honored to have been chosen as division head. I know that others of you could just as easily been chosen. Because we know each other so well, it may seem that we already know what each other thinks, but I want to take the opportunity that comes with a new beginning to ask us to think anew about where we want to go. So in that spirit I'll be meeting with each of you to get your ideas about what would advance our program. Because of our money woes, we do not have a new position now, but the chair has pledged support for a new faculty member next year and thus we can begin the planning for it now because recruitment takes a year anyway. We need to make a wise decision on this one so we need to think this through together.*

The speeches by external candidates make several crucial points: (1) I have a lot to learn (and by implication, I'm prepared to learn it from you). (2) I respect you and affirm your value, which I share, of excellence. (3) We're going to change. (4) There are no preconceptions; we'll look at the whole thing. (5) You'll be part of the plan. (6) I will pledge to help you survive and thrive.

The stump speech for the division head is modified because there is an internal candidate and because the group is so much smaller and has already defined, limited resources. But the tenor is the same: you will be included (I respect your opinions), we'll be moving forward, and we have something to look forward to.

Let's move forward with the dean as our example, though the processes are parallel for the chair or division head. In the same stump speech or in a succeeding one, she might say:

I know from talking to some of you during the search process that we need to add translational research to the clinical departments. At the same time, those decisions could have an impact on what we do in the basic science departments or on the kinds of people we recruit to our clinical departments. I'll be looking to you for confirmation of that and advice as to how exactly we do this.

This speech continues to keep open the possibility of their input. This is crucial, as this same "stump speech" forms the basis for further refinement of the idea. Think of it as a set of "successive clarifications" until a strategic plan emerges. The stump speech is really a transitional mechanism and precursor to a full strategic plan. It prompts dialogue that can help define the ultimate strategic plan and gets buy-in through the interactions and discussions it prompts.

Thus, the speech evolves:

I keep hearing the same ideas: translational research to begin in a division or two in the medicine department, probably cardiovascular and one other. The natural basic science partners seem to be pharmacology and genetics. Give me your thoughts.

To finally:

We're about to invest in the cardiovascular division of the department of medicine, pharmacology, and genetics. Any final comments before I pull the trigger?

What has happened is that the dean has moved from a bland, very open stump speech to an action item that will define her tenure as dean. Some will still object, but not because they haven't had a chance to have input. She has affirmed their values and clarified her own, and she has been able to test out some ideas and, in the process, gotten an idea of the resistances she will face.

While we believe that "meet and great" sessions are the most essential part of the process and yield the most data, there are various other means of learning about your new institution. Over the past 15–20 years, a number of consulting firms have offered services, ranging from financial assessments to evaluations of office staff—relative size, depth, and perceived competence. Such consulting services can also be tied to meeting general objectives, such as developing a strategic plan for consideration. Or you could use a faculty committee to develop the objectives of a strategic plan and then use a consulting firm to develop a business and implementation plan.

> As a general matter, faculty committees can be very useful. They need an appropriate charge, including critically whether they are advisory or decision-making, and the right membership to be effective, but used properly they can offer great value. After having had some meetings and determining an objective I might pursue, I would use a committee to flesh it out and put specifics on it. For example, after deciding we needed a review of the current research portfolio to decide whether we were prepared for emerging areas of science and to develop a set of priorities, I formed a research advisory committee to meet these goals.

To a large degree, the choice of what methods and how much of each to utilize depends on an assessment of your strengths and weaknesses. If you are more introverted, you might lean on questionnaires and outside consultants, as may those who prefer to make decisions by amassing large amounts of data. If you are comfortable with people and actually want to see their reactions (body language, affect, and the like), you will rely heavily on meet and greet.

> In my opinion, there must be some meet and greet. Faculty want to assess you, they want to see you respond to questions – does he sweat, is she defensive, can he think on his feet, is she mean etc. If you totally rely on questionnaires and consultants, you rob the faculty of that opportunity. As a result, faculty will see you as distant and aloof, and be cautious in providing you any useful feedback. They will want their input to be anonymous, just as you are. This is particularly true of deans and chairs, but perhaps less so for division heads.
>
> Of all these methods, there were two techniques that I used at UNC that yielded particular value.

Breakfast meetings. These are a form of "meet and greet." At the time of my appointment as dean at UNC, I set up a series of breakfast meetings with faculty. It was an open sign-up, and it was entirely voluntary. We met in groups of 8–12. The only rules were that no more than two members from one department were allowed at the same meeting. I imposed this limit because I wanted them to think beyond the department to what the school or academic medical center wanted to be.

The results were gratifying. Not only did they appreciate the opportunity to meet with me, but they especially appreciated meeting their peers in other departments and understanding their problems.

Later in my term, the troops became restless and I became aware of misgivings among the faculty. But none of my lieutenants could get a handle on the basis of their concerns. Neither could I, so I reinstituted a series of voluntary breakfast meetings to understand what was on people's minds.

Surveys. Because of the ease of electronic transmission, surveys of the faculty are relatively easy. At UNC, I used a modified Delphi procedure where we posed the question, "What would UNC be like if we were going to be the model medical school?" (Note: "Best" was not used because it invited comparisons to schools in the US News & World Report. We wanted to invite people to think out of the box.)

We received hundreds of answers, from a paragraph to several pages. In a Delphi procedure, you then take the responses and frame them into a series of options, return them to the faculty, and get them to vote on them.

I was amazed, not only by the volume of responses, but also by their quality. I didn't expect the answers they gave us. What was clear was that the faculty was first and foremost committed to the mission to serve the people of the state of North Carolina.

I must say I was astounded. I had spent my previous academic life at Duke and Emory, two fine private schools, but their faculties, if surveyed, would have responded with something like "to advance our knowledge of disease" or "to create the next generation of leaders." The scope would have been national, if not global, and the focus would have been to position themselves as number one.

That's not to say that one response is superior to the other. It's only to say that the ultimate values of the school serve as a starting point for all new initiatives. Change, which is difficult, becomes less difficult at UNC, e.g., if an initiative advances the school's mission, conflicts between contrasting value systems, such as subsidy vs. tub on one's own bottom, fall subject to the question of how they *affect mission*.

In the same vein, change at Emory or Duke is more easily accepted if it is seen as advancing the school's national position. Surveys are particularly useful in helping you elicit this information on values because they can encompass such a large group of people.

Summary

The first year should be an exciting year and should yield a surfeit of information. It is important to remember the two purposes at work here. The first is to amass relevant information. And the second is to start to shape the relationship that is at the heart of leadership: the leader–constituent interaction. You'll never get the opportunity again. We hope you will avoid rookie mistakes. By the end of the first year, most of the faculty will have formed an opinion about you. Did they make a mistake in picking you? Can they work with you? And most importantly, will they let you lead?

Chapter 8
Negotiation

When we teach our course on leadership development, we have learned that most faculty place negotiating at the top of the list of what they want to learn. When we survey them at the end of the course, they often list negotiation as the most useful thing they learned.

There are very good reasons for these answers. Your academic career begins with negotiating your compensation and start-up package. It's a rite of passage, but it often sets the limits of what you can accomplish as well. Further, as you move up the administrative ladder, your success depends directly on your ability to negotiate not just for yourself but also for your division, department, or school. It also depends on your ability to recruit others to your division, department, or school and to negotiate with them. You cannot find a faculty member who doesn't value hints on how to be a better negotiator. Further, you can hardly find faculty members who don't feel that they were "taken" in their first negotiation.

Learning how to negotiate is also the foundation for a whole host of additional skills, including recruiting (Chap. 9), conflict resolution (Chap. 10), persuasion (Chap. 11), making good decisions (Chap. 13), and stimulating change (Chap. 14). Each of these skills, which together comprise the toolbox of successful leaders, builds on the core principles that are honed in negotiating.

Despite the importance we assign to negotiating, when we reduce it to its elemental state, there are just four concepts to master. Everything else you may learn about negotiation can be viewed as simply an elaboration or refinement of these four principles.

They are the following: (1) there are generally just two approaches to negotiation—issue oriented and positional; (2) issue-oriented negotiation is the preferred approach in the AMC for a number of reasons; (3) maintaining and even enhancing the relationship with the person with whom you are negotiating are paramount; and (4) the core skill is the ability to elicit the other party's underlying interests and then to frame what you say in those terms.

© Springer International Publishing Switzerland 2015
J.L. Houpt et al., *Learning to Lead in the Academic Medical Center*,
DOI 10.1007/978-3-319-21260-9_8

There Are Just Two Approaches to Negotiation: Issue Oriented and Positional

I once read a book on how to buy Persian carpets. I learned about thread count, animal and vegetable dyes, as well as some of the classic designs. The last chapter was on how to haggle and get the best price.

Its methods were time worn and well known: don't accept the first price, be prepared to walk out the door and, and so forth. Not surprising, but its conclusion was if they accept your price, you've lost!

That's how it is with what Fisher and Ury call positional negotiation in their book, *Getting to Yes* [1]. In positional negotiation, the goal is to win; its methods include withholding information (hence the need for you to determine the thread count, dyes, and so forth on your own) and its assumption is that there is a fixed pie, a zero-sum game.

This is the mental model that most new faculty bring to their negotiation for their first position—and for good reason. Their experience in negotiating has been for a car or a house. Both almost always are positional negotiations.

But there is an alternative to positional negotiation. Fisher and Ury call it issue-oriented negotiation. It's the mirror image of positional negotiation. In issue-oriented negotiation, the goal is to find the best solution, not to win; its methods include sharing information and potential options, rather than concealing information. Engaging in these behaviors allows the pie to be enlarged in order to find the best solution.

Here is an example to clarify the difference. Let's say you are being offered your first academic job. In positional negotiation the chair will say: "I'll provide you a salary of $130K, 2 weeks of vacation, and funds for your travel to one meeting a year." If you respond that it is fine, or even if you decide to ask for more, such as $140K, 3 weeks of vacation, and two trips a year, you are engaged in positional negotiating or bargaining. It's no different from what you do when you buy a car.

In interest or issue-oriented negotiation for a first job, the chair would say this: "We're interested in you and think you have some real potential. I'd like to start by finding out what your interests, goals, and aspirations are and then share the goals and aspirations that I have for you. If we can find a common ground, I'd then like to tell you how we set salaries in the department, how I think you could fit in, and what our standard benefit package is."

Issue-Oriented Negotiation Is the Preferred Method in the AMC

You will find both types of negotiating styles represented in academic administrators. The issue-oriented style tends to work best because it creates and solidifies relationships, whereas positional styles are by their nature adversarial. This is problematic because the vast majority of negotiations are with organizational superiors—assistant professor to division head, division head to chair, chair to dean, dean to chancellor, etc. The authority differential is more easily neutralized if you can move to an issue-oriented discussion. In addition, you'll have to deal with these people again and again on a variety of issues.

For example, an entry-level assistant professor has almost no leverage in a positional negotiation. Chairs can capitalize on this by throwing out a salary number. The new faculty member's only recourse is to move the discussion to an issue-driven approach. If the entry-level assistant professor can move the discussion to how salaries are set and what he or she needs to do to get raises, the discussion will have moved to an issue-oriented rather than a positional discussion.

Further, if the one negotiating from an inferior position can find a common set of goals or interests, he or she can enlist the help of the one in the superior position. For example, assume the assistant professor was interested in translational research, which was also an interest of the chair. A simple statement from the assistant professor, "I think I can make a contribution to your interest in developing a translational research program in the department," can change the whole tone of the discussion.

> Shifting the focus to a shared group of interests actually removes the superior as opponent bargainer and instead enlists his or her assistance. As an administrator who has had innumerable faculty in my office negotiating with me, it is refreshing to find someone who is looking at the broader interests of the institution and what he or she can do to help move the place forward. Most cannot see beyond their myopic focus, and even were there a broader institutional interest, neither they nor I see it.

Maintaining the Relationship Is Paramount

No negotiation is ever won in the AMC if it alienates your boss. Thus, the first goal of any negotiation in the AMC is to maintain and even enhance the relationship. It is not about getting the most from the person with whom you negotiate. It's not like buying a used car where you want the best price. When you buy a car, you never need to see the salesperson again. Tough tactics in negotiating based on win/lose models are for these kinds of short-term, episodic relationships. Not so in academia. You need to continue to work with whomever you negotiate. If you are a faculty member negotiating for salary from a chair, for example, you need to leave his or her office with a good working relationship grounded in mutual respect. You will need to see him or her again. You will need more resources at a later time. You rarely if ever get enough resources in one negotiation. (We all know that everything costs twice as much as you think it does and takes twice as long.) And your promotion and career depend on his or her opinion of you. Don't blow the relationship over a few nickels or dimes.

The Core Skill Is the Ability to Elicit the Other Person's Underlying Interests

Without question, the best negotiators are those who can interview the other party and get to their underlying interests. But this is easier said than done. Some people are so entrenched in their positional world view that they can never be moved. However, you can be successful at this if you remember a few lessons about the art of negotiation.

You should begin your attempt to get to underlying interests by asking a series of open-ended questions: "What would you like to accomplish?" "What problem are we solving?"

You press forward by circling around with similar questions in order to clarify: "Help me understand where you are coming from." "What do you see this position accomplishing for you?" "I'm trying to be agnostic here, so help me understand why this is so important to you." "Could you share with me other possible solutions you considered or discarded?" "I'm prepared to compromise if I need to, but I can't if I don't understand what is vital to you out of all of this." "I think I got way ahead of myself by formulating a response without fully understanding your position, so can you help me with that?"

If you are fortunate enough to enter a negotiation at the beginning, you have a much easier time getting to interests. That is the case with the recruitment of a chair or faculty member. However, often you come to the table late in the process. Such is the case when the hospital director, for example, cuts your budget by 10 %. That decision is an action that is based on several prior inputs. The hospital has probably been working on its budget for months when you learn of your cut. Your cut of 10 % is the director's position, and you will never persuade him or her to do otherwise, if you cannot get to and correct those inputs.

Getting to those inputs is what negotiation is all about. To make the point another way, ask yourself when you are confronted with a position, say a hospital director who is cutting all budgets 10 %, what problem is he or she trying to solve by taking this position? Why 10 % and why across the board?

There are a series of questions that you might ask to get to these underlying interests. In the case of the hospital director above: "I know you've been putting this budget together for months now and probably the last thing you want to do is to review each and every input, but it'd help me sell it to my people if I could understand what the critical inputs were and how you got to them." "The budget is old to you but it's new to me and if I need to enforce it, I need to know the factors that led to this." Obviously, the sooner you can enter the process of a negotiation, the better.

Moving positional negotiators from their entrenched positions is not easy; sometimes they will hold on simply because they believe they have the upper hand. Other approaches may be needed in addition to simple, open-ended questions.

A different approach is to switch the discussion to your interests and ignore the positions that have been put forth. Say you are negotiating to buy a hospital for the healthcare system and a price is on the table as are several governance models. Instead of debating the specifics (positions), e.g., price, board seats, etc., you could just start thinking out loud about your underlying interests.

Let's step back. If we're buying this hospital, in order for me to sell this to my Board, we will need to be sure that we approve the budget and the strategic direction. We have to be sure we can make this financially viable and have enough control to do so, and we need a price that also makes it financially possible to succeed. What do you need out of this?

Another approach is to attack the underlying assumption of the zero-sum, win/lose game. Positional negotiators assume that it is a zero-sum game. They believe that anything that goes to you is taken from them. They neglect to think that there is another option. They fail to imagine a world in which you grow the pie and both benefit.

In the AMC, this is most easily seen in many interactions between the hospital financial officer and the department chair. The finance officer is focused on expenditures and costs and often therefore sees cuts as the surest way to meet budget. The chair is almost always interested in growth within his or her area and so wants to view potential revenues and growth as a way to meet budget.

These clashes occur regularly and keep a steady background atmosphere of conflict and discord in the air. Both sides come to believe that other side just doesn't get it. The finance officer offers homilies like "you can't spend money you don't have" or "the bank won't let you write checks if there is no balance," and the chair derisively refers to the finance officer as a "bean counter."

Growing the Pie

This example reflects two, nearly hard-wired, world views. One sees the world as finite. Opportunities are either in your favor or in someone else's favor, your first responsibility is to gather and then protect your resources, and you have a basic distrust of others' interest in you and a certain amount of pessimism. The second view is that we can all do better together than any of us can do alone, that people can be worked with and can work toward a common goal, and that they have a sense of optimism and believe there are opportunities out there that they just don't see yet. The first group follows a positional negotiating stance. The latter opt for an issue-oriented stance.

> My view is that faculty and administrators in academia enter the adult world in one of these two camps as their natural default position, but then adapt to the culture of the institution.
>
> When the naturally more optimistic individuals in the "make the pie bigger" camp are placed in a dog eat dog culture, they adapt to it but are vaguely unhappy with the lack of collegiality. Those who are disposed to be positional, when placed in a more collegial environment, take part cautiously at first and then gradually adapt. Several "convert" and begin to make career future choices based on whether the institution offers this open, collegial environment. Since I've seen the conversion, I believe it's worth the effort to move to a bigger pie stance. It certainly opens up the negotiation.

Successful negotiators know the difference between positional and issue-oriented negotiation, favor issue-oriented negotiation, know how to negotiate and still maintain relationships, and know how to steer the discussion to underlying interests.

The following vignette illustrates these four concepts.

Entry Job: Assistant Professor

Dr. White is a fellow in MFM in obstetrics and gynecology. She will finish her fellowship in a few months. She loves to teach and has started some interesting research in the lab for which she has been encouraged to apply for a K08 award. Her division head has encouraged her to pursue an academic career and arranged an interview for her with the chair to discuss it. Her fiancé is a fellow in another department with one more year left to finish, and so she would prefer to stay here for at least a year. She meets with the chair.

At the end of the discussion, the chair offers her a job as an assistant professor, clinical track, at a salary of $120K. She's expected to participate in call and do mostly clinical work, but the chair will support 20% time in the lab. She's really happy and says yes. In the course of the next few days, she learns that a man was brought in last year from another institution, and it's rumored he's paid $150K. She knows he doesn't take full call as she will have to, and she learns that he has 50% time in the lab. She has also been told that 20% time in the lab is not enough if she wants to launch a research career.

She suffers buyer's remorse and wants to go back and redo the deal.

What Should She Do?

Most people who read this for the first time gravitate to one of two poles. One group thinks she should go back and get it straightened out either because it's not fair or because if she didn't, she'd be angry all year. A second group thinks she should suck it up because she gave her word and should wait until next year to fix it.

And thus most people step into the trap. They take a group of propositions that are "positions," that is, salary, call time, etc., and start negotiating them. Instead, they should step back and wonder why the chair made that offer, what it says about his expectations of her, and yes, of course, what his underlying interests are.

The way we believe that this problem should be analyzed is to go back through what we just covered, keeping in mind the following points.

1. The difference between positional and issue-oriented negotiation: the positions are clear, $120K, call, etc. But the underlying interests are not. We know almost nothing about the chair's interests. For the assistant professor, we know some: the desire to stay in the area at least a year, an interest in teaching, maybe research

and patient care, but no overwhelming commitment to one over the other, at least, not yet.

2. A preference for issue-oriented negotiation: it's not clear if she knows her interests. If she is going to go back to him, she needs to determine what she really wants before she goes back to him.
3. The critical value of maintaining the relationship: she needs to think through how she will approach him and she needs to do some research about this other man who is making more and decide if there is a valid concern there or not. She needs to find a way to enhance the relationship with the chair while still getting her questions answered.
4. Identification of his interests: she needs to find a way to uncover the chair's underlying interests. She needs to do her homework, and importantly, she needs to ask him what his expectations and goals for the division and for her are.

Moreover, the relationship of Dr. White with her chair is all important. This is because her academic future depends on him and because she will need to go back a number of times over her career for more. But in this case, he will be making the really big decision NEXT year when she decides that both she and her fiancé will or will not stay. So for her, maintaining the relationship has to be paramount.

That reasoning may prompt her to do nothing, but it needn't.

The first "spat" in a relationship is all important because it sets the ground rules for ironing out differences. Rather than being a negative, it can be a positive because it begins to establish both your right to disagree and the process for working out disagreements.

> I personally liked having a disagreement when I recruited people because of that reason. I wanted to know how they would react earlier rather than later. I could always correct it early, i.e., not make the offer. It is much harder after they are hired. Then you need to go through a process of counseling, coaching, etc.

She will need to avoid positional bargaining, that is, "You offered me $120K, and I'd like $150K." Instead she needs to move the discussion to issues. "I realized after talking with you that I didn't really know the ground rules. I think I can do a better job if I know what you expect of me, how you'll evaluate me, what I need to do to be reappointed and how compensation will be determined, etc." In other words, she is asking for the rules of the game. She is trying to work this back to an issue-oriented negotiation.

If she is successful, she has a basis for future discussions, a clear knowledge of what is expected of her, and a basis by which to determine if what is offered to her both now and in the future is fair.

Some of you reading this vignette would be saying now "Wait! What about the obvious gender inequality?" That is certainly a legitimate concern. But in this case, it's added as a red herring to make a separate point. You know nothing about his background from the vignette. Let's assume he has an MD/PhD and a pink skeet on an R01 that indicates he's close to a funding level with proper modification of his grant. The point is added here purposely to remind people that negotiating on the basis of sameness is a very hard point to demonstrate. More frequently than not, people are not the same. Remember the difficulty with the null hypothesis: to prove that you are the same, you have to prove that you are no different in any respect.

If, for the moment though, we assume that these two people have the same qualifications and experience, then would we approach the chair on the basis of gender discrimination? Many would and we would understand, since establishing a basic sense of fairness and equality is important not only to the assistant professor but also to the morale of all faculty. However, we would generally counsel that her meeting with the chair should be set in a broader context, that is, the terms for the relationship, the rules of the game, etc. If she deals only with the gender issue, she hasn't set the terms of the relationship. She will have only established that there can be no gender differences without having established any of the other elements of the relationship.

She finds the chair very happy to explain his expectations for her, and his views are more robust than she had imagined. He had evaluated her as follows:

I see you as a potential long term faculty member. I realize that you and your fiancée may leave the area next year after you marry and he finishes his fellowship, so this first year is to see what happens. I have a major clinical need to fill this year which is what I want from you. I think that you might have an aptitude for research, and would be pleased if you moved in that direction. I am also willing to increase your release time to do research next year if you decide to stay and if you prove worthy of that investment based on what you do this year. However, you are considered an expert clinician and could be considered for a clinical role next year, again based on this year's performance and if you decide to stay in the area.

He also explained the salary of the MD/PhD for her. All of his formulations met her interests so they had a fit. They parted with the relationship strengthened, what she needed to know for this year, and how to plan with her fiancée for next year. This is a very successful negotiation, and it was accomplished by not jumping on positions but instead by getting the other party to talk about his interests.

Refinements to the Negotiation Concepts

If you can master the art of discerning underlying interests, you can be a successful negotiator. There are just a few refinements of the concept to keep in mind. The first is to know how to move from an understanding of interests to a completed negotiation.

Key Steps to a Successfully Completed Negotiation

The first step is identifying interests and then coming to an agreement on the common purposes to be accomplished, based on your understanding of interests. In the case of Dr. White, it is an agreement to use the year as a transitional one in which she uses some of the time to explore her research potential while furthering her clinical skills.

The second step is to operationalize it. In her case this means understanding how responsibilities, salary, and release time are set. In the case of recruiting a chair, it means determining positions, space, etc.

The third step is to set criteria to measure success. How will we know if we are successful? In the case of Dr. White, we can evaluate her progress toward a research career if she has preliminary data for a K award and has written parts of her proposal in a fundable way, as evaluated by experienced faculty in her department. Or her progress as a clinical faculty member can be determined by her ability to build a case load, her work units, and her reaching certain quality indicators for her specialty.

Parameters can be set in other contexts as well. In the case of a chair recruitment, each of his or her recruits can be evaluated. Those recruited to do independent research can be evaluated on their research funding, while clinical faculty can be evaluated on the basis of work units, caseload, and quality measures like Dr. White. Education can be evaluated in terms of what institution they match in their residency or with students based on student evaluations and standardized test scores.

The fourth step is to identify areas that are outside your control and that require help from others. This step is the one most often neglected in academia. It is also a common reason for failure. The idea is remarkably simple. If you want to build a sports medicine program, for example, you must have immediate access to radiology. If you want to build your surgery program, you must have adequate anesthesiology. If you want to build cardiology, you need coordinated efforts from EMT through the ER to the cath lab. Over and over again, efforts to build in these areas fail because the efforts of all parties are not engaged and ensured.

> I've seen this happen. I've been part of rebuilding a cardiology department that was already "rebuilt" before I got there; or a cancer center that had been rebuilt several times before. In each instance there are structural flaws that hadn't been addressed. Instead, a "new" leader is brought in to the same obstacles and he/she fails like their predecessor.

The problem stems from the mindset of the positional recruiter. They are going to hire you for the negotiated price, usually as low as possible - and look to you to fix the problems. If they understood their problems from a systems perspective with independent forces at work, they might spend more money the first time, but they could get it fixed the first time.

When Should I Negotiate and When Should I Not Negotiate?

The second refinement to the concept is to understand that sometimes it might not be best to open a negotiation. There is a term for this called BATNA or the "Best Alternative To a Negotiated Agreement" [1]. It implies that you should only enter into a negotiation when there is significant chance of improving your position. In the case of Dr. White, she should reopen the negotiation only if she can improve her position. If she returned as a positional negotiator, i.e., to get more salary or release time, it is questionable that she could have significantly improved her position, plus she would have the downside risk of alienating her boss. However, as an issue-oriented negotiator, she has a lot of upside. In an issue-oriented negotiation, she has a chance to learn the rules and to establish a relationship with her boss and secure his support. That is a huge upside and thus her BATNA would suggest that she should renegotiate.

When to Quit and Walk Away

We believe it's best to get what you need to be successful, but to leave something on the table. There is another negotiating term, ZOPA or the "Zone Of Potential Agreement," that should serve as a warning sign when you should take your foot off the gas a bit [2]. When you are close to your ZOPA, you might want to make one last pitch to close the deal. There may be a tendency to "get all you can," but we think it is more important in the AMC to not get a reputation of "taking no hostages" or being greedy. The reason again is the preservation of the relationship; you will be negotiating with that person again, and you don't want to start with the person feeling resentful because you humiliated him or her the last time. If you did, your current efforts will not prove successful. Always let the other negotiator save face and rescue something that they can point to as a victory.

Silence

Great negotiators use silence judiciously. People inherently attempt to fill silences. They are vacuums for other people's thoughts and words. If you can get your counterpart talking and filling silent spaces, you have a far better chance of finding out his or her interests. Silence often works better than your questions in eliciting valuable information.

Demeanor

Appropriate demeanor and emotional tone are crucial to successful negotiation but especially to maintaining the relationship. Don't ever try to negotiate with someone when you are angry at them. Don't get emotionally involved in the issue. You should be able to debate any issue from at least two sides. Practice your argument and then imagine the other person's best case and say it aloud to yourself. Take a detached, clinical view. Imagine yourself an anthropologist and observe the drama as it unfolds. You should enter the room with a smile and lightness about you and leave the same way.

Don't resort to ad hominem positions. Don't permit yourself to just say that they have a character problem. Force yourself to try and see the situation from their point of view.

Relate to the positive in everyone. Successful leaders (and successful people in general) find something to like in everybody. People know if you respect them or not. They will accept criticism, disagreement, and even decisions that hurt their position, if they know you respect them and their position, but they will rise up against you if they think you don't respect them. This point is also reflected in Chap. 6 on validating while listening and Chap. 7 on Getting Started the Right Way. Being respectful of those with whom you work should be obvious as a matter of civility, but it is also critical to your success.

References

1. Fisher R, Ury W. Getting to Yes. Penguin Books; 1983.
2. Spangler B. Zone of Possible Agreement (ZOPA). In: Burgess G, Burgess H, editors. Beyond intractability. Conflict information consortium. Boulder: University of Colorado; 2003. http://www.beyondintractability.org/essay/zopa.

Chapter 9
Recruitment: Negotiation in Action

The most important thing that a dean does is recruit chairs. The most important thing that a chair does is recruit faculty. Unless you can recruit you cannot build a great department or school. You can be the best manager in the world, but you can only take a B group to B+. You need an A group to get to A+.

And it's all about faculty. The best students follow the best faculty. The greatest successes in clinical work or research come from the best faculty. Building a great AMC depends first and foremost on the quality of the faculty.

We believe there are three aspects to successful recruiting. The first is to understand how using an issue-oriented model of negotiating leads to a very different outcome from using traditional positional negotiation. Using an issue-oriented method provides more and better information from which to make a good choice. Second, the goal is not just getting a person but rather getting the right person. Picking the right person, particularly for higher-level administrative positions like a chair or dean, involves looking beyond intellectual and technical competencies and creating a process that highlights a candidate's emotional and cultural competencies. And third, at all levels of recruitment, examining fit—both for the candidate and the institution—will improve your success in recruiting.

This chapter focuses on issue-oriented recruitment, which we believe is the best method of recruiting at all levels—faculty as well as leaders. In the final chapter of this book we take up the issue of picking the candidate with leadership potential and the role of fit, for the candidate and the institution.

Positional Versus Issue-Oriented Negotiation

The way that recruitment is commonly carried out involves positional negotiation. Usually, the recruiter (the dean or chair) charges a committee, and/or perhaps a search firm, and requests that three or so suitable candidates be put forward. The search committee typically begins with a "long list" and then, through a series of

© Springer International Publishing Switzerland 2015
J.L. Houpt et al., *Learning to Lead in the Academic Medical Center*,
DOI 10.1007/978-3-319-21260-9_9

interviews and vetting, comes up with a list of three or so. By this time, the candidates have been to campus and have given a seminar and talked with perhaps as many as 30 people. Then the recruiter picks the "best" candidate and begins to "negotiate." Usually, that takes the form of asking the candidate to send a letter listing "what it will take" to get him or her there.

The letter from the candidate follows, and the recruiter sends it to his or her administrative chief, who goes through the long "wish list" and writes "okay" or "can't do" by every item on the wish list. The recruiter and the candidate then go back and forth in a positional negotiation, until they agree or decide to quit and start again. We believe this method of negotiation is wrong in almost every respect from the point of view of getting the *right* person.

First, it establishes positional negotiation as the rule of the game. This creates the mind-set that every subsequent negotiation has the goal of getting as much as the individual can for himself or herself and the result of framing the discussion around that goal.

> Faculty members who return from visits where they are being recruited often tell me that they asked for twice what they needed. I ask them if they had a serious discussion about what they really needed or the obstacles or contingencies. They say, "No, but I won't get all that I ask for, so I asked for more."

Second, as the recruiter, if you follow the usual approach, you won't determine what the recruit wants to do with the department or, importantly, how the person prioritizes. A wish list approach tells you nothing. How the recruit decides what to do and what not to do tells you a great deal about the individual's analytic capacity and understanding of the department's culture. This is crucial data in figuring out beforehand if the recruit will succeed in your environment or not—if the person is in fact the best candidate.

And, finally, by using the "wish list" approach, you have no common agreement as to what you want the recruit to accomplish. Therefore, you have no way to evaluate whether the individual is meeting goals or not.

We believe that there is a better way to do this, which conforms to the model of an issue-oriented negotiation. Our alternative begins with the recruiter doing his or her homework on what the interests of the department are before the candidates arrive.

> One way to begin is by hiring a leader in the field to advise you. Say you are a dean and looking for a chair. You ask your department and you use your contacts to find out who is considered an opinion leader and sitting chair in that field, or recently retired chair. You invite him or her to come for a day. You make it as easy as possible to get your advisor to agree. All you want your advisor to do is meet with some of the faculty in the department, the search committee, and you as the recruiter and tell you his or her view of the following:
> 1. the national rank of the department; 2. its divisions with strong national standing and those without; 3. the market - how many other chairs are now open; 4. your advisor's ideas about what to do with this department if he or she were chair; and 5. if possible, potential candidates.

Using this approach, unlike the wish list scenario, you begin your recruitment with an idea of the department's national standing, some of its strengths and weaknesses, what needs to be done, the market place for chairs, and roughly how much it will cost.

Instead of staying in the background until the list of "finalists" is given to you, you as the recruiter should meet with all the short list candidates on each of their visits.

> In the first meeting you ask for their impressions of the department and whether they have any ideas yet as to what needs to be done to make it better. Their answer tells you a whole lot about the candidate. Does he or she have a plan before having gathered sufficient information? Is the person pretty good in sizing up the situation? How close does the candidate get to the expert consultant's assessment? Does the person show a respect for people? Is there an understanding yet of the culture or at least its importance? Using the "wish list" approach, you don't get any of this information.
>
> In the second interview you take up salary and refine the candidate's plan. By now he or she should be able to show you some insight and an approach as to how to proceed. The salary is taken up as a matter of fact. "How much do you make now?" You get the number and then I'd say something like "You should probably get a 15–20 % raise to take the job, so that'd be about x." Then, depending on the number, I'd say "We usually pay at the x AAMC percentile so that number would work", or if it didn't work, "That number would be out of line with the other chairs so we'll have to talk about this some more."
>
> This approach permits the recruiter to know the package, the direction that the candidate wants to take the department, how he/she deals with people, the salary and all one needs to know to make an offer. When the search committee presents a list, the recruiter can look at the list and know precisely what it will take to get each candidate, and pretty much who will come and who will not.

Determining the Size of the Package

If one follows the suggested issue-based model, the recruiter and the one who is recruited agree on what needs to be done, and then you put arithmetic to it. You break the objectives to be accomplished down into positions, whether MD, MD/PhD, or PhDs, and prices, both salary and start-up costs. You add in the salary of the person being recruited, plus administrative assistants, other staff, moving expenses and benefits, and so forth to come up with a number.

> This is relatively easy for the recruiter as he or she has done it many times before. But it can be a huge obstacle to the one being recruited, particularly if it this is the first experience being recruited. Certainly, I did not know this my first time, and most people who are looking at their first move have no idea either. So, if you are a first–time recruit, you need to seek a mentor to help you. If you trust the person with whom you are negotiating, you could even ask the individual if you might use his or her business manager to price the package. You could then double check this with your mentor and see how trustworthy the recruiter really is. The point is don't be ashamed of not knowing this. Nobody expects you to know this. Get help.
>
> As I became more accomplished as an issue oriented recruiter, I never had to review a "wish-list" letter. After the candidate and I had reached an agreement on objectives and broke that down into positions, I would tell him or her that I was going to send a draft letter that I believed reflected our conversation. My chief financial officer would then

draft a letter outlining every aspect of the discussion: objectives, positions, required space, promotion materials, fringe benefits, and whatever else we talked about. It would be marked very boldly "Draft". The candidate would then review it and make any additions or deletions. Usually it was accepted as is.

From Offer Letter to First-Year Evaluation

An additional advantage of determining common objectives during the recruitment is that those objectives become the basis of the person's review at year one. As mentioned in the paragraph above, the offer letter should include what it is that the candidate should be trying to accomplish. After a year, the letter is brought out and used to evaluate the individual's performance. The objectives are updated or altered based on a year's experience, and the new set of objectives becomes the basis of the following year's review. There is no question what the person should be doing and how his or her performance will be judged.

What to Do if the Package Is OK but Not Enough

Take the following example. An infectious disease faculty member is offered the position of division head at an institution that is attractive to him or her. The chair recruiting the individual wants the candidate to revitalize the research activities and in particular the NIH portfolio. The candidate researches the field and concludes that to accomplish what the chair wants, it will be necessary to fund five new positions. The chair does not disagree but responds that he can only fund two or three positions, depending on how rich the start-up packages are.

If the chair in this case were a positional negotiator, you would have no option but to press for three more positions and leave it at that. But, if the chair were an issue-oriented negotiator, you could respond accordingly: "You know, I really want this job and I'm in it for the long run. We both agree that five positions are needed to meet our goal. I understand also that this is a lot of money. How about if we do two or three positions in the first five years, and then, if I have a positive review at five years, we add the additional positions then. That will spread the cost out over ten years and that way we can meet our goal."

The point is that a too small offer may be the best that you can get. But if you can get the conversation into one with common and mutual goals, you might be able to meet the current cash flow availability but in the longer haul, get what you both want.

It should really be the responsibility of the seasoned recruiter to determine if the package is a realistic size. The first step is to set realistic objectives. If you are going to claim to aspire to be the top ten in something, you should be able to price what that will cost. If you can't afford it, don't set it as the objective. If a novice negotiator asks for too little, then, as the experienced one, you should tell the person so. "You know, I don't think that is enough to bring in three people."

Carry-Over Money

Most rookie negotiators don't consider the remaining funds in a package and whether they carry over. For example, let's say you were given start-up funds, and at the end of your 5 year term you haven't expended all of them. This is not an uncommon occurrence. In some institutions the funds are swept back to the recruiter and do not stay with the one recruited. As the one recruited, you want to ask for those funds up front.

> As the recruiter, I made a habit to raise the issue during the recruitment and offer carry over funds to the one I was recruiting. It was a positive sign of my interest in their success, and a positive factor in their decision. But it just makes sense given human behavior. Any time you threaten to take back unspent funds, the person goes on a buying spree and empties their account. If they control the funds, they are much more frugal, and don't have to come back to you to ask for more. It is also one more way to expand what might be a small package.

When You Are Carrying Out Several Searches at Once

It is not uncommon as a dean to be looking for two or three chairs at a time. This is when the issue-based approach outlined above really shines. Prior to the search, you invite in your expert and you anticipate what the costs will be. If you stick to your budget, you don't get into the trap of the positional negotiator who might spend all of the money in an effort to get the first candidate who comes through. You might decide to do two searches and delay one. The point is that by having a budget beforehand, you can make those decisions beforehand, and not after the fact. You can also tell candidates, "Look, I have three searches. This is the package—I can't do more—and as we discussed, it will let us accomplish our goals."

Some Additional Caveats on Recruiting

We would caution against allowing search committees to rank candidates. If a candidate hears that he or she is not the first candidate on the list, the person often drops out. Second, if the committee gives a number one ranking and that person is not picked, then the committee feels that they were not listened to. Third, you have more information than the department and the search committee because you've already negotiated the package.

You can say no. Saying "no" opens a whole new discussion and a way to see how the candidate will deal with not getting his or her way. A little spat on the way in can be helpful because you can see how they will respond in future situations when they're told no.

Many candidates get mentors to help them construct their wish list, and being schooled on positional negotiation, they ask for more than they will need. At other times, candidates will pick up long laundry lists of needs from the faculty in the department during the process of being interviewed. They then feel compelled to get everything to show the faculty or mentor that they will be good leaders. In both instances, going back to actual needs based on an issue-oriented negotiation is the only way to save the recruitment. If they come to believe that they need to get what their mentor thought they should get, or what the department wants, you will lose them.

You make mistakes when you get lazy. You should make your own calls to vet candidates. They may be to people in important positions whom you do not know well or to those you can call friends. Of the two, friends give the best advice by far. Some feel a call to the dean or chair of the school from which you are recruiting a candidate is both courteous and useful. However, those calls can be misleading because self-interest can kick in, and they tell you what they want you to hear. It is more useful to call friends. They have your interests at heart. This also is considered in more detail in the final chapter.

Being desperate is the next problem. If there are no viable internal candidates and if the external field is weak, you become desperate and just pick somebody to fill the position. That is almost always a mistake. It's like going to the grocery store to buy food when you're hungry. You always buy something you don't really need. Here you may want to consider closing the search, naming an interim for a year or so, and then going back a year later.

> Always recruit the family. Candidates make family decisions. At one place I interviewed the recruiter left my wife, who had her own career, in the hotel and suggested she visit a tourist attraction that day. At another place, the recruiter had arranged several valuable meetings in her field. We went to the second place. I've lost candidates because their children would not agree to move. The point is the family is not something you consider as you get down to the final points in the negotiation. It should be a major part of any negotiation and dealt with in the first visit.
>
> Pay attention to whoever you use as a realtor. A simple negative comment about the school system, for example, can lose a candidate. We always used realtors that one of us in the dean's office had used ourselves and prompted them that the school systems would be an important issue if we anticipated that it would be.

Go out to dinner together. Go out with your partner, the recruit, and his or her partner. A social setting provides information you might not otherwise discover. It helps to spot stiff or absent social skills and to see whether the person has a sense of humor. It also gives you information as to how comfortable recruits are with people in a social setting and whether they honor the partner's opinion or just listen to their own point of view. It is also an opportunity for you as the recruiter to check in and see how their day went and if they need to see different people the next day.

> Look for a sense of humor. Humor is a high level adaptive mechanism and when used properly it doesn't degrade others, it lacks hostility, and it shows comfort in displaying one's weaknesses. There are a lot of things going right from a psychological perspective if people

have humor. You can survive picking people without much humor, but it makes life easier if a candidate has a good sense of humor.

Recruiting should be fun and not adversarial. It's an opportunity to meet the best and the brightest in a field. The reality is that the recruiter and the recruited are mutually dependent on each other. My final line to each candidate I decided to pursue was, "I only succeed if you succeed, so come here and we'll make it work."

Chapter 10
Conflict Resolution: Making Friends with Conflict

What drains people the most in AMC leadership positions is dealing with interpersonal conflict. It results in burnout, leads people to resign, and is a major reason why good people don't want to take these jobs. Offer any novice groups of deans, chairs, or division heads a leadership course and ask them what they want covered, and they will say the same thing: first, negotiation and then how to manage difficult faculty or how to supervise poor performers. Ask any retiring cohort of leaders in an AMC what was the hardest part of the job and they will say managing difficult people.

There are many reasons for these views that have already been outlined in this book: the myriad and conflicting values and world views of the faculty and staff, the nature of authority, the culture of independence, and the ideal of equality and free speech. Nobody salutes; people need to be brought along to buy into new ideas. Passive aggression is too easily a default position; too many are narcissistic.

Unfortunately, many leaders respond to resistance and disagreement in nonproductive ways that only make the situation worse. Often, the first response is anger and actions based on anger. The leader may use the anger to confront the offending person, but in an excessive fashion. The leader then embarrasses himself or herself and gives the other person a legitimate complaint about the way he or she was treated. This becomes the issue, and the offending behavior cannot be addressed for fear of retaliation.

Another favorite response is the ad hominem attack where the issue over which there is a disagreement is discarded in favor of an attack on the personality or character—"that person is just lazy" or "passive aggressive" or "greedy" or "narcissistic." Or the leader leans on the vertical hierarchies and tries to impose his or her will from above. In addition to not working, this behavior has the added effect of lowering the esteem in which the leader is held.

But there is an alternative. You need to make friends with conflict and become comfortable with people who disagree or resist. There is too much conflict out there at an individual, departmental, and institutional level for it ever to be completely resolved. Conflict need not to be dreaded; it needs to be seen as omnipresent and part and parcel of the creative process.

© Springer International Publishing Switzerland 2015
J.L. Houpt et al., *Learning to Lead in the Academic Medical Center*,
DOI 10.1007/978-3-319-21260-9_10

Moreover, most conflict should just be ignored. There is no reason to wade into it. Your job is not to convert people to your sociopolitical view. Democrats and Republicans or capitalists and socialists can work together in the workplace. People also don't have to embrace your every idea. Don't expect a big "hooray" for each and every initiative. Don't expect these people to be your therapist and hold your hand. It's enough to get sufficient support to get the particular job done.

You should only deal with conflict when it interferes with the work of the institution going forward. The leader's preoccupation should be with clearing the obstacles to work getting done. Disagreements that create background noise but don't stop the work going forward should just be ignored. If you are thinking of stepping in, there are five questions to answer before you attempt to mediate a conflict.

1. What are the interests of the parties involved in the conflict and what are yours and those of the institution?

Here we are drawing on the same methodology as we do in negotiation generally. The core skill is your ability to understand the true underlying interests of all parties. The best negotiators can get to interests just as the best conflict resolvers do. Miss on the interests and you'll miss on the resolution.

2. What are the personality issues of the parties involved?

We're not looking for a personality diagnosis here, but instead an understanding of characteristics. Is the person a big picture or a detail person, narcissist/big-ego type or not, rigid or compromiser, zero-sum-game type or big-pie type, a person with causes, etc.? You should know these answers from your contacts with the person over time and use them in deciding your course of action and strategy.

3. What are the political pressures?

This includes peer groups, important external people (the mafia as we've called them), other issues under consideration at the time, etc.

4. What is the right process?

If you are in an institution that values process, then how you do what you do is as important as what you do. You need to touch all the right bases, involve the right people, and take the time to follow that process. If you work in a more executive environment, you can move more quickly. You still need to get advice and consult widely enough to get buy in, but then you can just proceed.

5. Am I in control of my feelings?

Never attempt to work out a conflict when you are angry with the person. Get beyond all your feelings and view conflict resolution dispassionately. See it as chess match or a negotiation exercise. Approach it clinically, with equanimity and without emotion.

Dr. I.M. Special: The Difficult Personality

You are the chair of medicine. You were just approached by one of your prize assistant professors to ask you to intervene with Dr. Special.

Dr. Special is an older professor, who was already a professor when you were an assistant professor in the department. He has an excellent reputation and indeed spends much time "waving the flag" away from the department at various meetings and AMCs around the country. He is in much demand because early in his career he did some interesting research, is an electrifying speaker, and has an uncanny ability to market himself. He has held forth at Board of Visitors meeting and has appeared on the local TV station. He travels in the highest social circle locally and counts members of the Board of Trustees among his patients.

While he is brilliant in his own curmudgeonly way, he demeans young colleagues, often blows up at staff because he feels it's "their job" to do whatever he asks of them, and has a track record of being unable to collaborate with anyone. Recently, his bad behavior seems to be increasing, as staff have complained about his abusive verbal behavior and administrative assistants have refused to work with him. One has brought a grievance against him. The medical director complains that he refuses to sign his charts, and now an assistant professor claims she should be the first author on a paper on which Dr. Special is demanding to be first author.

He has been tolerated for years because he brings national standing to the department and because he is a celebrity outside the department and so "connected." To the local mafia, he is the face of the department.

However, the escalation of the behavior, the willingness of younger staff members to voice complaints and bring a grievance against him, and the complaint by the assistant professor leads you to think that you have to do something. What would you do?

In teaching our classes, two different approaches are usually taken. The first is to focus on his "connections," and the severity of his personality disorder, and to decide that little can be done. This leads this group to favor a very limited approach. A second group are visibly annoyed at his poor citizenship, which would "eat like a cancer" at the group's morale. They feel that he needs to be removed. They are never sure how to do that though.

On the surface, either seems reasonable enough, but both jump the gun a bit. The first focuses exclusively on politics and the second on personality/behavior. A more reasoned approach takes into account both but also takes into account the interests of the institution, as well as other parties, and the process to be put into place to accomplish the desired outcome.

The Interests of the Parties

To go back to our most fundamental question, what are the interests of the parties involved? What are Dr. Special's interests? What are your interests as the chair of medicine? And, most importantly, what are the interests of the department?

There are several parties involved—Dr. Special, the assistant professor, the administrative assistant who brought the grievance, you as the chair, and the other faculty who are watching this drama unfold. The only way to find out what their interests are is to interview them.

We'd start with the assistant professor and then the administrative assistant before seeing Dr. Special.

Let's assume the following: With respect to the assistant professor, she did the work, including the data collection and analysis and the original writing. Dr. Special was her collaborator and they talked about the study before she started the work. She says he was away most of the time and didn't regularly check in with her. Her interest is in getting a first-authored paper as she works toward promotion.

The administrative assistant says he would berate her and at times yell at her, "What don't you get about x or y?" She says that no one else behaves this way and asks why he should be allowed to do so. "He's been doing it for years and getting away with it." Her interest is in just not having to deal with him.

With respect to Dr. Special, we don't know what his interests are. We'd suppose that he wants to be a celebrity, but maybe he also wants to be above the "law"—that is, the spoken and unspoken rules of behavior and decency in the department. Being a celebrity is not a problem, but being above the rules for behavior could be. You talk with Dr. Special, and he is a little amused over this tempest. "Yea, I might have raised my voice once-hasn't everybody?" With respect to his charts, "No problem. I've just been out of town." On the subject of the assistant professor, "It's a misunderstanding on her part—it was my research idea. Yes she collected the data but a research assistant could do that and yes she wrote the first draft but that was how I was teaching her to write papers. Further, she's entitled and overvalues herself and this is further proof of that". He ends the interview with "Are we done? I've got things to do." After speaking with him, it seems clear that he doesn't see any problem in his behavior. His interests are in being left alone to do whatever he has done in the past.

For the rest of the department, they're divided. The older ones say that they are used to him and just don't count on him for anything. In the past he's gotten a little out of control but he can tamp it down for a while and probably will even though he won't admit to anything. The younger ones find him boorish and not charming at all. They think he's a virus and don't know why he should be permitted to be exempt from the normal rules of behavior. They want you to show him that his behavior is not okay. The interests of the department, at least for the younger faculty, are in establishing values of civility, fairness, and equity.

Your interests are in establishing your authority and norms for behavior in your department. Your job is to provide a safe and productive environment. You need to decide if this behavior is outside the bounds. You ask yourself whether you should encourage a Darwinian environment where people need to fend for themselves or a more protective one with definitions of civility.

Personality Issues

Dr. Special probably is narcissistic and has some common features of personality disorders—it's not his fault; he's not to blame; it's not anxiety provoking to him; it's others who have the anxiety. He's an example of one who demeans those below him but charms those above him. For years it didn't affect the work of the department, but now it does. The assistant professor is affected in doing her work at the least, as well as the administrative staff, and the morale of the younger faculty members suffers.

Political Pressures

There are significant ones outside the department. Any reprimand or penalty could be shared with those important people, who could potentially call the dean, and result in your hearing from the dean.

The Correct Process

You've taken the right first step by talking to the interested parties. Given the political pressures above, you'll need to discuss with the dean whatever you decide before carrying it out. The rule for those above you in the organization is no surprises.

If You're Not Angry, You're Good to Decide What to Do

What to do revolves around the issue of culture and values. Are the prevailing norms the pursuit of stars, rankings, and Darwinism, or are they equality, collegiality, civility, and care and feeding? Observing the prevailing norms is important because there will be no challenge to your authority if your decision is consistent with norms. It will be business as usual.

However, there is an added wrinkle in this case. Here the older and younger faculty are split. The older faculty are used to Dr. Special's behavior. One explanation is that it could be in keeping with older norms of stars, rankings, Darwinism, etc. In addition or alternatively, their indifference could represent the erosion of older norms of civility, collegiality, and so forth. Gardner has commented that values tend to decay over time and periodically need to be renewed [1].

Meanwhile, the younger faculty want a stance taken against Dr. Special's behavior and, by implication, are asking for a new set of norms—equality, collegiality, civility, and care and feeding. This whole new tide of thinking may have nothing to do with the department's past but may have to do with generational issues. Generational issues often introduce new values that are at war with older ones and cause conflict between the older and younger members in a department.

Thus, the ante has been raised. The question may no longer be what the prevailing norms are but whether the conflict can be used to change the culture to a new set of values.

This question is much more to the point than the two alternatives outlined by most classes we've taught (limited vs. wholesale approach). Also, the answer to this question gives you the starting point for how to act. This is why you need to go through the discipline of asking what the interests are. There is no one answer to this question. This is what leadership is about—coming to a defensible position when there is more than a single choice. Given the personality and politics, is this a threat to values and is the opportunity to change the norms important enough to do something? Further, given the personality and politics, what would you do?

The first possible choice is this: to decide whether the department, institution, and dean are committed to rankings, stars, and a culture of Darwinism. In that case, you "go with the flow" and reestablish the status quo. You separate the administrative assistant from Dr. Special and tell him to sign his charts (actually you probably don't tell him anything; you just e-mail the medical director that Dr. Special has been out of town and has assured you that he will be signing his charts) and tell the assistant professor that she's a grown-up and has to work it out with Dr. Special.

The second possible choice is this: to decide that this is an opportunity to change to (or rediscover à la Gardner) the values of collegiality, civility, and care and feeding. You have decided that the department has been eating its young, that this has to stop, and that recruiting the brightest and best in this world requires a more welcoming and civilized culture. In this case, you might develop the following strategy.

You begin by meeting with the dean and telling him what you are about to do and why.

Then you meet with Dr. Special and tell him how much he has contributed to the department and how much you are all in his debt for putting the department on the map. With regard to the charts, you are pleased with his response and have explained to the medical director that he was away and would be signing his charts going forward. He quickly interrupts to say he has already done it. You say "great. But on the other two issues, I've decided to go a different way from just ignoring them because after talking to a good number of the faculty, I believe there are important issues here."

"The first is that there is a perception that we are eating our young - maybe in the old days we could get away with that, but now we need to grow our young to replenish our faculty. Moreover, our ability to recruit requires that we be seen as more nourishing. Look, the world has changed and we need to change with it."

"I hope I can count on your support and leadership to assist me in this. Now, what I've decided to do is this...." This sequence is important because you want him to know that this is not a negotiation, but that he can climb on board and save face, i.e., that he doesn't need to be embarrassed, but you've decided and the train is leaving the station.

"First of all, I'm going to ask a group of senior members of the department to look at the issue of first authorship. We all know there are guidelines about this, and so this is not an issue for bartering. Secondly, I think you should apologize to the administrative assistant at whom you yelled. I will separate you and you won't have to work together, but I think you owe her an apology, and I've told her that."

The way this has been handled doesn't require his acquiescence. Whether he apologizes or not doesn't matter. What does matter is that the department knows that you took him on by (1) forming the committee and (2) noting that you think he owes the administrative assistant an apology. Had you demanded that he apologize, you would have set up a power struggle that he could win by not doing so. By simply telling her that you think he owes her an apology, you haven't demanded anything nor have you given him a way to win a power struggle. But in these two moves, you've taken steps that will become known publicly and will establish the new rules as well as your leadership.

This case demonstrates the two-step process that we believe is necessary to resolve conflict. It's impossible to get it done in one meeting.

> If you try to combine letting the person present his side and delivering a verdict all at one time, my experience is that it does not work. First, the person assumes that you had made your mind up before you met with him or her and nothing that he or she said mattered. The second reason is that the person always presents countless new pieces of data that challenge your case. Thus, I prefer collecting all the data in one or more meetings before making my decision so I know all of the challenges and the person knows that I have considered them. Then schedule another meeting for the verdict.

Reference

1. Gardner J. On leadership. New York: Free Press; 1990.

Chapter 11
Mastering the Art of Persuasion

> Leadership is the process of persuasion or example by which an individual (or leadership team) induces a group to pursue objectives held by the leader or shared by the leader and his or her followers. Gardner [1].

Gardner's view of leadership is consistent with the premises of this book. Faculty decide first of all whether to bestow authority on the leader and then if they're going to follow him or her. Getting from an initial bestowal of authority to having a group pursue a set of objectives is the art of persuasion. So central is persuasion to Gardner that he equates it with leadership.

This chapter outlines a framework for learning to be more persuasive within the AMC. It draws on several concepts already covered in this book. The central idea is that persuasion requires an ability to elicit others' interests and builds on the lessons learned in Chap. 8 on Negotiating and Chap. 10 on Conflict Resolution: Making Friends with Conflict. It also requires an understanding of groups and what is expected of the leader, of the role of culture and values in determining what's acceptable, of how to fashion your message to the existing norms, and of your personality and its strengths and weaknesses and how to utilize them most effectively.

The second part of this chapter teaches how to narrow the area of conflict or differences, the virtues of brevity in being persuasive, and the importance of framing your argument in terms of the interests of the larger institution.

A final section focuses on persuasion as it specifically applies to fund-raising.

On the subject of persuasion in general, it's easiest to begin by talking about what persuasion is not. It's not asking permission to do something, and it's not doing only those things for which there is consensus. So much of this book thus far has emphasized bringing along the group to a consensus, seeking input broadly, and shaping a common vision. It's important to clarify that the process doesn't stop there. Those processes are vital but are frequently not enough. You don't always get agreement. You need to push forward when the group can't get to conclusions themselves because of split allegiances. You need to be capable of persuading them to take the next step.

© Springer International Publishing Switzerland 2015
J.L. Houpt et al., *Learning to Lead in the Academic Medical Center*,
DOI 10.1007/978-3-319-21260-9_11

Persuasion is also not a sign of weakness. On the contrary, persuasion is a forceful process that is a necessary step in effecting any change. It takes intestinal fortitude and the willingness to assume the risk of ridicule, which is a course only the courageous pursue. Those lacking courage just release ultimatums. Persuasion is not for the wimpy.

Finally, being good as a persuader has very little to do with smooth oratorical delivery. How you make your case, how you frame the issues, whether your message resonates with your previous actions, whether it reflects listening on your part and includes the group's ideas, and whether it has the institution's interests at heart are determinative of the outcome than the smoothness of your delivery.

Let's try these concepts out. *You are the chair of a research-intensive medicine department. Your department is running in the red. The dean and hospital director hire a well-established consulting firm to delve into the problem and suggest a solution. A long report follows with all sorts of graphs and national benchmarks, but its suggestions boil down to two: faculty salaries need to be trimmed by 10% overall and faculty need to increase productivity by 10% to reach the black. The report is sent to the faculty, and the chair of medicine is trying to determine his or her strategy.*

You begin by asking these two related questions: (1) what are the interests of the group(s) and (2) what are the values at play? The groups have to include at least the department, the hospital, the school, and the individual faculty members. The interests of the school and hospital are clear. They want a balanced budget, and they want the department to stand on its own bottom without a subsidy. This is a clear statement of values-a reflection of the particular culture. It is not clear from the vignette if the school or hospital would provide stimulus money to jump-start new programs going forward, but the operating budget needs to be balanced.

The school, however, has additional interests. Assuming that this is a research-intensive school, the department of medicine traditionally leads the way in research funding for the clinical departments and usually for all departments. Since the stature and standing of a research-intensive school depend on its total research funding, any change that might diminish the department of medicine's research productivity would lower the rank of the school and even the university. Thus, the school needs to assess the effect on research funding.

The faculty have a vested interest in their careers and therefore anything that affects teaching, research, or patient care. They respond that the "bean counters" have taken over. Nothing in the entire report focuses on either the educational or research mission. While the consultants might argue that they focused only on the financial issues, their utter insensitivity in terms of not mentioning research or education only confirms the faculty's fears that the heathens are at the gate. Thus, the faculty start believing that this pathway is not in their best interest. Further, since it is generally accepted that research needs subsidy, they believe they need (deserve) to be subsidized. Finally, they read the report as saying that they are being lazy. Yet they believe they work longer hours than any hospital administrator and the raft of associate deans in the dean's office. In short, they're angry.

Since you know the different parties' interests, you can now develop a strategy to respond to the report. Based on concepts covered earlier in this book, you begin by asking these questions.

Does my plan demonstrate my interest in the group—all the subgroups or just one—and does it demonstrate my commitment to the survival, betterment, and success of the group? Does it support the core values of the group and is it consistent with the values I've demonstrated before?

You begin to fashion a statement based on these questions. You decide to embrace the intent of the consultation but distance yourself from the report itself.

"I know that many of you are just a little angry that the report mentions nothing of our academic mission and focuses only on clinical productivity. I can't help that. It was done by a group of consultants who were paid to focus only on the financial side. We are going to have to do the bridging and the hard work of seeing how this fits our academic mission.

Second, there is no getting around that the school wants us to run a balanced operating budget, so we are going to have look at whatever we do within that context. Several of you have pointed out to me that the report doesn't look at start-up and seed funding, so I will be trying to clarify this with the dean's office at some point. I'm not going to start there because it will look like a knee jerk response and possibly whining, so we'll begin with our own analyses of salary cuts and workload.

But stay with me. We'll look for a way to come out of this that preserves our mission, or at least we'll tell you what it will take to get out of this with our mission intact. I'll be meeting with the division heads to work through this and then we will get back to you. Any questions?"

You have spoken to the most pressing issues—your role as leader to protect their interests and to sustain the values that underlie your department. With that done, you will then want to ask yourself a couple of further questions: Has authority been bestowed on you already and are you using your personality strengths in deciding how to roll out this initiative?

You clearly would prefer to take on something of this importance only after your authority has been bestowed. However, sometimes these events are thrust on you before that can occur. In that case, you must take it on anyway because the value proposition is vital to the department. If it does come early, just be sure that you use an open process that permits maximal input.

With regard to personality, we have suggested that all of us have to work around our weaknesses and play to our strengths. To use introversion and extraversion as an example, the chair who is an extravert might go to each division by division and talk this through. The introvert on the other hand might send out an email to division heads outlining the problem, inviting feedback to be sent to another person, who would collate the responses—perhaps a vice chair for clinical affairs—and promise to get back to them. He or she might then call a meeting of the division heads with the feedback and his or her analysis in hand. Both would be acceptable and in keeping with their personality.

In the meantime, the chair is meeting with the dean. For the purposes of this exercise, let's say that the chair extracts a promise from the dean of start-up packages for two new recruits but no ongoing salary support. You conclude that you need to increase productivity to 12 %, rather than 10 %, using the additional 2 % for their ongoing support. Also, as a result of your talking with the division heads, you decide to distribute the salary decreases based on productivity or lack thereof, rather than across the board.

You ask the division heads to preview this with their faculty and then call a faculty meeting and you say something to this effect:

"We have a plan that I believe is doable and that meets our objectives. It provides for a balanced operating budget, but it also permits us to keep our missions intact. It includes two new positions. The dean has agreed to fund two new recruits but the department must carry the ongoing costs. To accomplish all of this we need to increase productivity by 12% and we will need to trim 10% from our operating budget. The division heads and I have decided not to do across the board cuts but to do it on the basis of individual productivity. We used national benchmarks to come to those decisions. Thus some will see a little change and others will see more, but we believe using these standards will be more equitable."

This story represents a strategy for being persuasive. It begins with interests and the values that underlie the plan. It includes their concerns and still responds to the dean/ hospital director. It is consistent with their culture, and it offers hope and a "way out." Even though it calls for more sacrifice, it doesn't matter. What's the difference between 10 and a 12 % increase in productivity? Not much, if it reaffirms the core values of the group. Ten percent is a lot if it comes with an abrogation of the core values; 12 % doesn't seem too much if it affirms core values. As we said earlier, culture is king.

We offer three further suggestions to enhance persuasiveness.

Shape the Message to Diminish the Areas of Conflict

As you work with the division heads, you are constantly shaping the message (as in Chap. 7 on Getting Started the Right Way) and narrowing the field of disagreement. Good persuaders narrow the field of disagreement as much as possible. In the case described above, you can imagine areas of agreement (protecting mission, treating divisions differently, cuts based on productivity, using national benchmarks, and getting the dean to kick in). You can anticipate disagreements emerging with the final distribution of salary cuts and productivity numbers. This is fine. You have narrowed the field of disagreement, and at this point you step in. "We've been through a long process, we agreed on this, this, and this, but some are still concerned whether the numbers are right. I am convinced that all have been heard, and that the overall mission of the department is protected, and that further discussion will afford no more agreement, so we're going to go with this plan. I'm open to reviewing it in a year's time to see if it is fair and meets our goals. I especially want to thank the committee, etc."

The result of this statement is that arguments by naysayers against the plan are harder to make. If someone wants to argue against it, he or she needs to take on the areas of agreement—the mission and the division heads' choice to base reductions on productivity and national benchmarks. It would be a hard argument to win simply on the basis of personally being disadvantaged.

Practice the Art of Brevity: Sentence, Paragraph, and Page

The most common mistake people make when asking for something or trying to persuade is to talk too much. When you meet with your boss to request something, or when you meet someone in a hallway to whom you must make your point, or when after a long discussion you are driving home your point, you need to be brief.

Imagine this scene repeated numerous times in the course of a day. A faculty member is meeting with his or her chair with the hope of securing some more resources. The faculty member starts talking, gaining more and more passion with each line, as he or she launches into a long, but perfectly reasoned argument as to why his or her idea is the best thing since sliced bread. Meanwhile, the chair is trying to seem interested and makes special efforts not to look bored but is wondering where this monologue is going. After some time has passed, the chair interrupts and takes over the conversation by asking questions.

In the end, the faculty member fails in his or her attempt. As they part each other's company, the chair is thinking, "Ask that person the time, and he or she tells you how to build a clock." *Meanwhile, the faculty member is muttering,* "The chair has a two minute attention span.... He or she has ADHD."

There are obvious reasons for this miscommunication. Faculty members often make their living by asking previously unasked questions and by then answering them. Researchers make a living by asking questions and finding new, clever ways to answer them. Shortcuts to that process are seen as superficial. Psychiatrists ask more and more divergent questions or ask for endless clarification, to address a problem in psychotherapy. Internists are drawn to complexity and may seek even more information to answer a question.

On the other hand, many surgeons and emergency room doctors seem to be wired differently. They routinely are required to make decisions on less than complete information. And so are chairs, deans, provosts, and presidents. They make decisions to fund things or not, based on a set of priorities determined long before a particular faculty member enters the room. For them, the decision to fund the idea or not is based more on how this proposal fits his or her priorities than the brilliance of the presentation. Consequently, they need less information to make the decision.

This same dynamic occurs in conversations between chairs and deans, between deans and provosts or presidents, and between anyone talking to a potential donor. And all result in lost opportunities unless one can make a case in a sentence, paragraph, or page.

As hard as it seems at times to get this across to those of us in academia, we are already expert in this process. We just need to apply it. We all know what a topic sentence is.

All of us have written abstracts—that's a paragraph or two. And all of us know how to write a one pager. We just need to break easy habits and practice.

The process is easy. You begin by stating your case in a sentence. You pause and look to see if your audience is still interested, and you give them a chance to speak. If they don't respond, you move on to your paragraph, which essentially buttresses your argument. Then you stop and wait for their response. If they don't, you continue to your one-page description. But be sure to tell them what you want right out of the box—don't keep them guessing.

> I had learned that a very influential State Senator had accompanied his wife and was in our chemotherapy infusion center. I walked down to meet him to find him sitting on the floor because he had given his chair to the family in the next cubicle. The place was packed, and he was not the only one sitting on the floor. The overcrowding was magnified by the fact that it was in a building 50 years old and the ceiling was 7 feet in height.
>
> After talking to him and his wife for a while, I invited him to take a walk. I was intent to show him the new hospital wing we had just built. Once we got outside, he said, "That's a disgrace. The people of the State should not be treated in that space". I thought for a millisecond wondering if I should respond that we had spent $5 million over the past three years trying to doll it up - but that was defensive and irrelevant. So I said," You're right. It needs to be replaced" (note: a sentence). I waited and he seemed to nod to go on. "It's an old TB hospital, built 50 years ago - it can't be fixed, the ceilings are too low, the hallways too narrow, and the floors can't handle our new heavy equipment" (a paragraph).
>
> He began to ask questions: "why don't you replace it then" to which I said "we're tapped out after building the new neuroscience hospital, the women's hospital, and the new children's hospital. We're in debt to the tune of $400 million plus dollars". He asked "how much would it cost?" I responded - "I don't know for sure -we'd need an architect and engineering firm to be sure, but my building person says about $110-130 million". He said: "Get me the numbers. But it has to be done right. The people of the State deserve better".
>
> We ended up with a $210 million hospital with an attached physician office building. I'd never suggest that all efforts would turn out so well, nor that it would have happened if it weren't justified by follow up detailed presentations. But I am convinced the sentence, paragraph, page approach works. You need to catch their attention, to place a foot in the door. One of the faculty, a division head, who took our course tried this in his budget hearings with his chair and reported the following. *"The budget meetings were scheduled for 30 minutes each. Everyone before me went over. I was finished in 17 minutes and out of there in 22 minutes and got everything I asked for! The others didn't".*

We believe the crucial ingredient is to pause. When you pause after a sentence or paragraph, you are inviting the other person to ask questions. If they start asking questions, they take over the discussion and begin to shape the discussion. In time, they begin to take ownership. If you never pause, they never have that opportunity.

Always Look to the Interests of the Larger Institution; Try to Make the Pie Bigger

A single faculty member is going to be more successful if he or she brings an idea forward for funding that benefits not just him or her but other faculty as well. A chair is going to be more successful if he or she recommends a program that benefits another department as well as his or her own. A dean will be more successful in getting institutional support for a program that benefits more than the school.

> In about the year 2000, the University of North Carolina invested extensively in a program in genomics. The idea started with the faculty. Both the School of Medicine and the College of Arts and Sciences had faculty engaged in strategic planning processes in

parallel. Independently, both concluded that their first priority was a program in genomics. Thus the initial thrust was spearheaded by the two largest schools of the university. The initial argument was that the two schools with the largest number of grants have identified a program on the cutting edge of science, which in order to remain a leader, the university needed to invest in.

At about the same time, our argument received a boost when the national press began writing about genetics and the "age of biology." Genomics was touted as a tool by which agriculture and medicine would move forward. This added validation and a sense of urgency to our message. We added to our argument, "We can't sit out this dance."

Our next step was to see if other schools wanted in on the effort. Quickly, the Schools of Public Health, Pharmacy, Dentistry, Nursing, and Library and Information Science signed on. We now had a pan-university initiative.

At this time, the university had an interim chancellor, who had been a very successful businessman. He called me one day for a "litmus" test. He asked, "How many of the deans are prepared to put their money in this, and how much?" I sent out an email message and the deans responded within four hours. They all were willing to contribute. That same day he had his answer.

Ultimately it fell to the newly named permanent chancellor to approve the program. He did his due diligence, and the program was funded.

This story plays out again and again. The department of microbiology wants to develop an immunology center. It has a much better chance if pulmonary, asthma, pediatrics, and perhaps others are in from the beginning. Want a cosmetic surgery initiative? Include not just plastic surgery, but ENT, dermatology, and ophthalmology.

There's a good reason for this. There are always limited resources. If a program request comes forward that benefits more than one person or more than one department or more than one school, it's much more likely be funded because it "raises all boats." The pie getting bigger is a powerful argument.

A Special Word About Fund-Raising

When it comes to fund-raising and dealing with a donor, brevity does not work. In these instances, your willingness to give generously of your time and thoughts is a major part of the persuasion process. It is best illustrated with an example.

I flew to the potential donor's city. Our development officer had already flown in the day before and had dinner with the potential donor. We arranged to meet at the airport in a private room. The development officer accompanied him. I flew in and had arranged to fly back out in about two hours.

I told him that I'd like to tell him about the school and what I was trying to accomplish, but I wanted to learn about him and his interests as well. (I always try to set an agenda at first and get their input so that I know that I'm going where they want to go.)

He said "great", so I asked him if he wanted to start. I told him what I knew about him and asked him to tell me more. He seemed willing to start and he began the usual biographical sketch - where he grew up, his parents, where he went to school, and his career. Some talk of their marriage and kids, and others don't. How much detail they go into doesn't matter. What I do is mirror what they say and fill in my own history - in the same detail. We often find common backgrounds, attitudes, beliefs, etc. But that doesn't matter either. If we don't, we remark how different our paths were.

Then I launch into a discussion of the school - its size, its faculty, students, programs and so forth. I tailor it to what I heard him express but not entirely. I learned early on in fundraising to never assume what the other's persons interests are, at least not until they tell you themselves. (In one of my first efforts at fundraising, my development officer set me up to talk to a potential donor who had made one gift to our cancer center to ask for a second larger gift. As I was building momentum for "the ask" she interrupted me and said "Jeff, I gave a gift in honor of my husband to your cancer program. That's all. What I'm really interested in is Alzheimer's. We have it all over our family".) So I keep it open until the donor makes his or her decision and tells me. We continue with the discussion with the school, and I answer his questions. At the end, I might ask if anything I covered interested him. In this case, he said, "cardiology". So I asked him if he'd like to meet one of our leading cardiologists and talk further. If he has no particular interests yet, I just ask to meet with him again - perhaps in my office - and offer to give him a tour of the medical center.

The point is that this is a process of relationship building and can't be hurried. It's still a matter of persuasion. What the donor is doing is trying to determine if you can be trusted to use his or her money wisely. That judgment is totally on his or her schedule.

Here are a few other lessons I have learned. They may prove useful to you.

1. Don't conclude that you are poor at fundraising if you are unsuccessful the first time, for at least two reasons. First, some causes are harder to raise money for than others. When I was the chair of psychiatry I felt I was awful as a fundraiser, and I was quite concerned that when I became a dean I would be unsuccessful. Fortunately that didn't prove to be true. I learned that raising money in psychiatry is very hard, because most people with severe mental illness do not have a lot of money. Those who have money and an interest are usually parents of disturbed children, and most do not want to memorialize their situation.

The second reason relates to your pool of potential donors. As dean I had access to several donors and I could match them with their interests. As a psychiatry chair, I didn't have that access or the ability to mix and match. I see many chairs who feel defeated because they can't raise money. Don't give up; it's not always easy at that level, and your lack of success may not be a problem with you. Keep soldiering on.

2. Get over your fear of asking. The wealthy are going to give their money somewhere so it might as well be you. I meet people who fear "the ask", like it matters if they are turned down. Get over it.

3. I have no evidence for this except my experience but it seems to me that there are two kinds of money out there, each of which requires its own approach. The first is old money - money that was earned in another generation, and is still being distributed. The second is new money - money that was made by the donor you are working with. For older money, a charity has likely been picked - cancer, children, etc. - often with guidelines that future generations follow. Your approach is to meet those guidelines, not to try to get them to go outside their guidelines.

However, for people who made their own money, the approach is different. Often the money was made in financial services or the tech world, although some may have come from manufacturing. They are entrepreneurial. They want to know the return on investment, the deliverables, and the timelines. The approach here is to treat them like a business partner and work out a business plan together. You also need to help them define their areas of interest.

In closing, I offer one further observation about persuasion. Of all the people I've seen or worked with, two individuals stand out to me as the best. While they follow the rules we've outlined here, there are two more characteristics that they share. First, they all practice their speech spontaneously. I'll be talking to them about some topic, and the issue that is currently bothering them, sometimes not even related to the subject of our discussion, comes up. When it does, they begin practicing a speech that they anticipate having to give some audience of what they want to do. They look for feedback. They refine it in front of me. I didn't ask them for a speech - they just start in. And I'm sure they do it with others. I believe they practice and practice their speech. These people are so good, and even though it's an N of two, I offer the lesson for your consideration. Practice might make perfect.

The second thing I noticed about these two people is that they don't rely exclusively on logic or data. One of them is a master of the metaphor, while the second uses anecdotes, adages, or witticisms. Their arguments are warm, humorous, and down to earth. They entertain and enthrall you. Their level of skill may be beyond many of us, but the power of anecdote and metaphor, with just enough data, is more persuasive to me than data alone.

Reference

1. Gardner J. On leadership. New York: Free Press; 1990.

Chapter 12
Running a Meeting

Sample the opinions of faculty or division heads, chairs, or deans about group meetings, and you'll hear the same chorus of negative responses:

"It was a waste of time and I have so much work to do"; *(after a meeting)* "what was that about"; *(from a retired chair to his successor)* "I'll do whatever you want except I won't go to another meeting"; *(to someone who missed a meeting)* "you didn't miss anything."

At the same time, we insist on doing much of our business in group settings. And there are many good reasons for this. We value wide input, we expect to be included in decisions, we value transparency, and we like to hear ourselves talk. So we do business in groups, and we shouldn't expect any change in that soon.

While most of the negative comments above speak to the issue of efficiency, there are other reasons to be concerned about doing business in groups. Groups can become irrational and provide the setting for bad decisions unless they are kept on task. Keeping them on track is the subject of this chapter.

But first, a digression by a psychiatrist. In my training we had experiences in Tavistock style groups. These are two-day long, psychoanalytically oriented group exercises where the group leader only comments on the process of what he sees but says nothing to guide the group solve problems. If some members go off on a nearly psychotic bent, the leader makes no comment or suggestion that the group challenge it. When placed in this environment for two days, the group can become more and more disorganized, offering aberrant solutions to problems. In one such group exercise, the group was tasked to find a way to join with and merge with a second group. In a group without leadership someone will emerge and take over the group. In this particular exercise, after two days of frustration and the deadline bearing down on them, the leader who emerged suggested kidnapping a member of the other group, and from a position of strength, negotiating the merger of the groups. And they did. After the experience was over, the group members were chagrined at their behavior. These were professional people. They couldn't believe that they assented to such a strategy. But they did, while under the influence of a group with a leader who did not direct, did not reality-test, and did not keep the group on task.

My take home message was that groups can support aberrant behavior in the absence of leadership.

© Springer International Publishing Switzerland 2015
J.L. Houpt et al., *Learning to Lead in the Academic Medical Center*,
DOI 10.1007/978-3-319-21260-9_12

I've seen similar things in AMC meetings. Somehow without good group leadership, the loudest, most reactionary scheme can take center stage.

So we begin there. The fundamental task of the leader is to help the group do its work. Yes, he or she must stimulate a wide discussion but must also bring the group together as they develop a consensus. The process is the same as we outlined in the section on diminishing the areas of conflict (Chap. 11). You should define the task, and as you find areas of agreement, capture that land, then redefine the new territory, and gradually work down to the smallest area of controversy. Here is one example.

You are chairing a meeting considering a faculty member for tenure who worked in the lab of one of your distinguished scientists. He was a postdoc and then stayed on as an assistant professor and is now up for tenure. The group likes his work, the publications are in first-rate journals, but the question of his independence from his mentor is unclear. After a while, some of the group go back and open up questions that seem to have been settled, which they'd rather do than deal with the area of controversy. Rather than let this deteriorate, you intervene and say the obvious: "It seems we agree on the quality of the science, his national standing, his record of funding, and his meeting our criteria, save for the issue of independence." *In this way, you have just captured the areas of agreement and taken them off the table and have defined the remaining area to consider, thus narrowing the area of debate and defining the work that the group still needs to do. You may go on:* "Let's have a straw vote and find out how many are concerned enough that we need to investigate further and how many think we know enough to go to the final vote." *Whatever the vote, you have a decision and can move forward.*

This does NOT mean that you talk a lot. If you are the group leader, you give up the opportunity to pontificate. Instead you need to encourage the group to talk and use their statements to pull together a plan. In this way, you can frame areas of agreement by using the very points made by members of the group. If you choose to do all the talking, the group will rebel and do nothing that you wish.

Aids to Keeping Groups on Task and on Time

Keeping a group on task and on time requires the leader to know the purpose of the group discussion and to remind the group of what the purpose is. In academic settings, the purpose is usually one of three: (1) to share information, (2) to make a decision, or (3) to have a discussion without a decision. At any one time the leader needs to keep the group informed as to what the task is right now. "I've asked Joe to give you an update on xyz – we don't need action on it." Or "I've asked Joe to give you an update on xyz and we're going to want your feedback because we will be coming back at another time for your vote on it." Or "We're going to vote on xyz today. We've brought it to you several times for discussion, and we'd like to bring it to closure today. I've asked Joe to summarize the discussion so far and to put forth a motion for your approval."

A written agenda helps keep the group focused. If it's a small, informal meeting, the leader should begin by orally announcing the agenda. Otherwise, a written one is necessary. Here's one example:

AGENDA	
Department X meeting	
1. Approval of the minutes	**Randal Brown**
2. For information (20 min):	
Update on healthcare reform	**Mary White (10 min)**
Update from committee on resident education	**Jack Frost (10 min)**
3. For discussion:	
Expansion of medical school to new counties	**Jennifer Green (10 min)**
4. For decision (20 min):	
Promotion of JG to associate professor with tenure	
Offer to MG as assistant professor, clinical track	
5. New business	

As you introduce each topic, you reiterate the purpose ("this is just for discussion, or we will need a vote here, etc."). The times in parentheses are optional, but you tell the speakers before the meeting how long you expect each of them to speak.

Some Common Problems and Potential Responses for the Group Leader

1. Nobody talks. "It's very important that we get your opinion because we're going to make a decision on this shortly. Joe – you start if off, what's your opinion?"
2. One person dominates. "Thank you. Now I need to hear from others." *(If you need to do so, call on someone.)*
3. People are talking, but no new information is being offered and people are just repeating themselves. "We seem to have come to a common point. Are there any dissenting opinions? This is important because we don't want to shortchange ourselves. Are there any further thoughts, no matter how contrarian or even seemingly stupid?"
4. You're not hearing your own point of view or views you know are held by people in the group. "You know I expected to hear x or I know that in separate discussion some of you have expressed y."
5. A contrarian expresses a diametrically opposite view to where the group is now.

There are a variety of approaches, depending on your diagnosis of the situation. First, you should always see if there is a kernel of truth in what has just been stated. It's said that even in paranoid delusions, there is a kernel of truth. Look for it. On the other hand, there is the anti-leader, that is, the person who wishes to usurp your leadership position. You should challenge this effort in some way. To do so, you might use the group: "Does anyone want to pursue this?" If there is no response from the group, you might say: "Good people can disagree; let's go on from where we were." Or you might use just the line: "Good people can disagree," without involving the group. Sometimes the contrarian is just a person with a cause and works his or her cause into every discussion. In this case it's just a diversion and not a threat to you as leader. You might say: "You know I agree with that, but it's a discussion for another day."

Having Influence in a Group and Getting Your Voice Heard

1. Pick your seat/raise your hand. The position where you sit is essential. Sitting and facing the leader or sitting at the end of the table so you have a full view of the participants gives you an advantage in getting your voice heard. If your voice is weak and you can't force your way in with a loud voice, remember that you can always raise your hand when someone is speaking. The chair of the group will call on you.
2. Try being the summarizer. If you choose to summarize the discussion, particularly at the end, you can set the agenda for the group. The summarizer of necessity screens information, and if it is coherent, this person's summary can become the collective memory. It's an easy step from there to suggest the next issue for discussion.
3. Or, be the gap filler, that is, the person who says what is not being said. The gap filler is very influential, because groups tend to avoid the most important issues unless they are reminded. The gap filler leads to a more balanced view. For example, picture a workforce discussion where the group is arguing for more physicians: "I haven't heard us talk about physician distribution. There's no doctor shortage in our counties."

Before the Group Ends, When You Are the Group Leader...

As chair, make sure you summarize the decisions and next steps or ask someone else to. If a member of the group spontaneously does so and you agree, just say something like "that summarizes our discussion" and thank him or her. If it is lacking, add what needs to added.

Whoever takes the minutes ultimately sets the policy agenda because people rarely remember anything else. So monitor minute taking. Also if you are on a national group and asked to keep minutes, you just might want to do it. You'll have more influence than you might otherwise have.

After the Group

A weasel comes into your office after the meeting and wants to massage/continue/ reform the committee debate. If you disagree with the weasel and agree with the group, you should say something like: "You should have spoken up. A vote of 14 for and 1 against is not a veto" or "You're asking me to gut the entire authority of the group. Why should they meet and spend their valuable time, only to have you stop me after the meeting and reverse what they did?"

If no decision was made, you must invite him or her to bring it up next time. Let's assume that you agree with the weasel. "You know I have some sympathy for your opinion; you'll have to get it into the discussion next time." Then next time you should use the line: "Since the last meeting, I heard some other views voiced" and call on that person, *but if a decision was made:* "you know, you should have spoken up. You'll have to ask the group to reconsider next time."

Or after a meeting, a mole appears in your office. Remember that not all moles are bad. It's a good way to get information out. Nothing spreads faster than a rumor. But if the leaks can't be tolerated, you might confront the group and ask them for ideas as to how to proceed. If all else fails, disband the group and start over.

Summary

Becoming an expert group leader takes practice but can be very rewarding, not only for you but also for the group. A superior group leader gains all the advantages of the group—transparency, involvement, and diverse viewpoints—and also makes good decisions.

If you want to become better, our advice would be this. Rehash the meeting immediately afterward with a close circle of advisors who have some emotional intelligence and look for the underlying themes that ran through the meeting. Discuss together alternative approaches to what you said and did. This is especially important for those of you who are a little low on the emotional intelligence scale.

Chapter 13
Making Good Decisions

The surest way to succeed is to string together a series of good decisions. But what is a good decision? Generally, the judgment that a decision is good takes some time to let all of its consequences—good, bad, and unintended—play out. Thus, it's hard to say whether a decision is good at the time it's made. Yet no organization can move forward without someone making decisions in the present.

So where do you turn to learn about what constitutes a good decision? One way to approach the problem is to consider whether there are any characteristics that good decision-makers have and seem to share and whether there are common mistakes that poor decision-makers share. If there are, what are they, and what can we learn from them?

Based on our experience, though admittedly limited, we have settled on four characteristics that good decision-makers seem to share: First, good decision-makers take into account personality and political factors. They see them as part of the issue but not the whole issue, whereas poor decision-makers base their decisions solely on political or personality factors or fail to factor them in at all.

Second, good decision-makers have a natural propensity to act, but they also have a sense of timing or tempo. They are neither too slow nor too fast at deciding. Third, they always have the institution's interests at heart, rather than self-interest. Fourth, good decision-makers learn from experience and get better over time, whereas poor decision-makers don't seem to do so.

We expand on each of these.

© Springer International Publishing Switzerland 2015
J.L. Houpt et al., *Learning to Lead in the Academic Medical Center*,
DOI 10.1007/978-3-319-21260-9_13

Personality and Politics Are Part of the Issue but Not the Whole Issue

We proposed an algorithm in the chapters on negotiating and conflict resolution. It is this: take a problem and subtract out the political and personality factors in order to find the *ideal* solution, and then add back in the political factors and personality factors to get the *best possible* solution.

You will find some leaders who will focus solely on the political factors and solve all problems from that perspective. But if that is how you decide, you are a politician and not an institutional leader because the best possible decision is not always the political one. Others focus solely on personality factors and act as psychologists rather than as institutional leaders. Decisions made on this basis are also not usually the best ones and have the additional downside of empowering the personality disordered by allowing them to have a significant impact on outcomes.

The best leaders can both assess the political and personality factors and decide when to act. They understand first and foremost that the best interests of the institution are not always served by following only personality or political dimensions, though they do factor them in. Recall the case of Dr. Special in Chap. 10 on Conflict.

Finally, sometimes no decision is the best decision. In these cases, the political and/or personality factors are so great and the relative benefit so small that it is not worth taking action.

Having an Urge to Act Is Important but So Is Tempo

Collins used the term an "urge to act" [1]. Decisions require a natural tendency to wade into conflict rather than a starting point of conflict avoidance. Good decision-makers don't have to overcome a fear of acting.

> It's my view that these people who act are not immune to anxiety, nor do they fail to weigh the risk. Instead they have an override that tells them they must do this. I've talked with people I consider great leaders, and they confirm these points in many different ways. "I didn't want all those battles but I just had to protect the company;" "It's my job ... it comes with the territory;" "How could you face yourself in the mirror each morning if you ran from that;" and "You've got to play the cards you're dealt."

But timing is also critical. Decision-making can be too fast or too slow. On one end of the spectrum, you may encounter the hyperactive leader, flitting from one decision to another. We know the consequences of this approach: an organization lurching in one direction and then another, with the leader reacting to the crisis du jour and leaving people wondering what's next. Their approach is ready, fire, aim.

On the other end of the spectrum are those who are passive. For them, every potential decision needs to be studied further or one more committee needs to bless it. Their habit is ready, aim, aim, and aim again. We've all lived with these leaders and we know these consequences. In addition to endless committees, there are reports that aren't acted on. Moreover, there is a culture where things can't get resolved, so the same problem is continually faced; nothing ever happens.

The "too fast" decider may appear to make decisions so quickly that no one believes that they were consulted or that their opinion mattered. This problem is addressed in Chap. 6 on Emotional Intelligence, in the section on Validating While Listening.

As a stop gap measure, too fast decision-makers need to adopt the habit of not allowing themselves to make a decision the first time a problem arises. They need to take a week. In that period of time, they can sleep on it and consult with others, which they should do even if they don't think they need to. Even if they don't change their mind, it will at least *appear* to others that they are deliberative.

The approach if you are too slow or too passive about decision-making is more complex. It's useful for you to understand the tangible benefits of exercising authority. First, it defines who you are. Your initial decisions begin a trail of behaviors that will, in the end, lay open your values and character and define your legacy. Once you make enough decisions in your term, you will not need to explain your philosophy and vision. They will be evident in your trail of decisions.

Second, once you've established your values by a series of decisions, it makes future decisions easier to explain as long as they are consistent with your previous values/decisions. This means that the early decisions may need more explanation than later ones. It also means that you need to explicitly tie the earlier decisions to your values. The discussion later in this chapter on "early decisions" is an example of such an approach.

Third, decisions solidify your authority and define your power. The old adage holds: use it or lose it! A person in a leadership position who avoids or, even worse, appears to run from a decision will lose the allegiance of the group and thus the group's willingness to follow future decisions. On the other hand, once the person shows an ability to make decisions, it becomes known that there is a new leader in town. People find it reassuring. Someone is capable of asserting control.

For the "too slow" decision-maker. I believe that the inability to make decisions is due to two personality factors. The first is conflict aversion, and the second is perfectionism.

The conflict averse leader is usually afraid of displeasing people. These people shy away from conflict because it raises their anxiety level too high. They'd rather not act than become subject to disapproval. The problem is that avoiding making a decision brings disapproval as well. The facts are that even "win-win" decisions will disappoint someone. Other decisions will disappoint many. One of my superiors once said to me as I was seeking his advice on what to do, "Jeff, I figure a good decision angers 1/3 of the people, pleases about 1/3 of the people, and 1/3 just don't care." In addition to the problem of paralysis, the conflict averse can be manipulated by advisors. With just a suggestion that an influential person will be upset with a decision, the conflict adverse will not pursue it. All that advisors need to do is suggest someone's disapproval, and they can get their way.

The second cause for inaction that I see is perfectionism. This is another defense against anxiety. Here the need is to do things perfectly so as to win approval, and, hence, to do nothing unless absolutely convinced that their decision is perfect. This causes a far too drawn-out decision process.

Moreover, most decisions are made without complete information. It's not that we don't use the information we have, it's just that the information is not available. Will a new program in cardiology break even in three years? Will a new recruit get his or her grant in year two? We can't know for a certainty. It's inevitable that you might make a bad decision. This is intolerable to the perfectionist. You must be able to make decisions with less than complete information.

It is very difficult to change people who are conflict adverse or perfectionist. You can appeal to their sense of duty that the institution needs them to step up, or point out that if they don't act, someone else will decide the matter for them. You can work on ways to mitigate the negative backlash or try to convince them that the backlash will blow over. Or you can try the tips in Chap. 4 on Personality for handling the perfectionist.

But in our experience, a better approach is what we call the alter ego approach. The idea is that every leader has strengths and weaknesses. It's not a big deal if you aren't perfect. But the truly great leaders compensate by putting people on their leadership team that make up for their weaknesses. This is the concept of collective competence that we addressed earlier. We've seen that the addition of one person to a leadership team alters the dynamic in a way that the leader becomes more decisive. Some leaders just get a sense of security when a respected ally joins with them in making a decision. The ally infuses the leader or the leadership team with confidence.

While it is easier to slow down the too fast deciders than it is to speed up the slow, the fast deciders get into trouble more quickly and thus may not survive long enough to correct their ways. On the other hand, slow deciders often last long periods of time because fewer decisions mean fewer divisive decisions and less active opposition.

Good Decision-Makers Have the Institution's Interests at Heart

This is a key principle in Collins' distinction between Level 4 and Level 5 leaders [1], and it is discussed in Chap. 6 on Emotional Intelligence.

Good Decision-Makers Get Better Over Time

It seems that many people grow wiser as they mature and age. This is particularly true of those who are willing to learn from experience, by asking themselves whether they could have done things better. We expect people to learn from their mistakes and become wiser.

In the spirit that we can learn from our mistakes and become wiser, I offer some tricks that I believe have made me a better decision-maker. Here are five that I've learned over time:

1. Background noise. Not every issue that someone thinks is important is important. One of the hardest things to learn is how to distinguish between issues that need to be addressed and background noise. These environments we work in are never going to be conflict free, nor are people going to stop complaining. For example, faculty are never

going to be completely pleased with the equity of teaching or committee assignments, or the functioning of the billing office in the practice plan, or the efficiency and user friendliness of the grants office, or the speed of response of the technology transfer office. Your job is to try to ferret out those issues that are real problems that you need to address and those that just reflect dissatisfaction despite the reasonable assignment of teaching or committee responsibilities or despite an adequate set of services, even if they are not up to the hopes of the faculty. Sometimes deciding not to act is the prudent course and not a symptom of conflict aversion.

2. Respond to the issue, not the person's emotion. I remember fondly the faculty member who taught me this lesson. She was a distinguished professor, but she was critical and curmudgeonly. Many walked on eggshells around her. She came into my office and began carrying on about this issue and that. I began trying to piece together some kind of response when she broke off my conversation and said: "Jeff, I don't expect you to fix this today. I just want you to listen."

Of course, she was easy on me. Most who will come to see you are not only anxious and hyper-caffeinated but also are demanding that certain things happen. But the same lesson applies. Respond to the issue, not to the person's emotion. From that time forward, I became even more cautious when I felt that people were dumping their emotions on me. Some people have a remarkable capacity to come in and leave you with their anxiety, their anger, or their despair. Don't pick up their baggage or their urgency.

Over the years I learned to end these session with summarizing what I heard them tell me, and then "I'll need to sleep on this" or "I'll need to consult with a few people and I'll get back to you" (and specify if it might be a few days or longer).

3. Don't always try to be the first. There are many examples in the past 15 years of the academic medical center where letting others take the lead has paid off.

The first academic medical centers to employ primary care physicians in a network in order to create referral lines lost their shirts. They employed physicians previously in private practice, promised them a full salary to bring their practice with them, and then watched as these physicians "retired" while at work.

Promised a full salary, the physicians had no incentive to work hard. Many of these networks had to be disassembled; the physicians bought out and transferred back to private practice. The second iteration of this idea worked: the physicians were paid on a strict incentive basis.

Good leaders know when to lead and when to let others take the lead. The drive to lead in everything belies an inability to set priorities. You can always sit out a dance.

4. Understand the difference between low-hanging fruit and third rail issues. Low-hanging fruit represents decisions where there is near unanimity on the need to move forward. These decisions usually benefit the group in a way that is clearly understood in material terms, i.e., more salary or space, or removing an obstacle, such as improving the efficiency of the grants office. Such decisions usually come about because of a change in external circumstances that opens up an opportunity not available before. These require little strategy and are easy to implement.

On the other hand, third rail issues are those that violate the will of the majority of the group, or for which there is major disagreement within the group. They usually involve the perceived loss of resources (e.g., a new tax) or the violation of a major value of the group (e.g., granting tenure to clinicians with weak publication records). They require a well-thought-out strategy, which is taken up in the next chapter.

5. Don't win the battle but lose the war. Some battles can't be won or are too costly. Winning a battle over the budget that advantages you in the present but sours all future negotiation is a pyrrhic victory. Repeated negotiation is the rule in the academy. The dean returns to the president repeatedly, the chair to the dean, and the division head to the chair. Consequently, your relationship to others is paramount. Winning any battle that threatens the relationship warrants very cautious consideration. Pick your battles.

The Special Circumstance of the Novice Leader
and the First Decisions

The first decisions you make go a long way in assisting the faculty in defining who you are and in determining whether they wish to entrust their future and that of the institution to you. As we said earlier, your decisions begin a trail of behaviors that will, in the end, reveal your values and character and define your legacy. Often, the first decisions will be forced on you. You will be in the midst of your meet and greet when issues of retention or budget or some other crisis will arise, requiring your action. Some will be small, and some will be significant. You don't find them, they'll find you.

Think of these first decisions as teaching moments. Use them to send a message. If the first decision is thrust upon you, and it's not the one you would choose to introduce yourself, welcome it anyway. Analyze the message it sends and the values it implies. If you are blessed with an early quiescent period, pick the decision you want to introduce yourself.

Take as an example a new surgery chair. *The hospital director asks that he or she increase throughput on the operating room. As a first decision, the new chair reassigns operating room time, taking it from underperforming senior members of the department and giving it to more productive younger faculty. This decision is made after the faculty has been consulted and an analysis of the culture completed. It was viewed as a decision that had to be made, and the new chair decided "let's do it now rather than later."* What more needs to be said about Darwinism for that department?

Sometimes when first decisions are forced on you, they may be so complicated that you can't give them a thorough consultation with the faulty.

> In my first month at UNC, a distinguished professor met with me to say that he had a recruitment offer from a prestigious school and would leave if I didn't provide him with more space. He pointed out that there was adjacent space to his that was underutilized and that housed an unfunded investigator from another department.
>
> I checked. He was right about the adjacent space. In addition, the professor seeking the space was highly funded; he already had more space than most in absolute terms, but in funded research per foot, he was "under-spaced."
>
> I would have liked to have had time to have the faculty study the space issue, but the delay might have meant losing a really good person. I also knew that one of my prime tests was going to be finding funding for building new research space. However, that process, even if successful, would take 4 or 5 years. I also knew that UNC culture required faculty input, fairness, and equity among faculty, but also that there was impatience by the "high producers" because of a sense that they were subsidizing the "low producers."
>
> Further, I had concluded through my visits with the search committee that I was going to have to move the institution more in the direction of the high producers' wish to be rewarded for their productivity. I viewed my task in this problem as regenerating (in Gardner's word discussed earlier [2]) the value of meritocracy. However, I had not yet earned the faculty's trust, so any decision would be premature.
>
> Ironically, I saw this as easy. No matter what I did, I didn't have the buy-in, so regardless of my decision, I'd offend some. So I went with my values, seizing an opportunity to

let the community know what I stood for. I announced that I was going to take the underutilized space and retain the valued professor. I went on to form a faculty committee to work out the details by which space would be reassigned, e.g. how long unfunded space could be fallow, the process for requesting space, and so forth. In the end, one of my signature accomplishments was the creation of a space policy ratified by the executive committees of the medical school and the creation of a committee comprised of faculty and dean's staff to manage space.

First decisions open you up to your first negative reactions and introduce you to Monday morning quarterbacking. You need to learn how to deal with these. They come with the position. I found no magic wand here to make negative publicity go away. And I came to the most simplistic of resolves to deal with it. First, did they understand what I did? If they got it right, that is, what I decided and why I did it, I usually did nothing, even if they didn't like it. If, on the other hand, they either didn't get it right or they misinterpreted my intentions or values, I corrected it. In the end, you need to live or die on your record. You just want to make sure the faculty get the record straight.

Taking a Stand: Value-Driven Leadership

We have acknowledged earlier that stated core values are sometimes just given lip service and that people recite them but often are consumed with self-interest or misplaced institutional loyalty and avoid taking stands beyond lip service. But the simple lesson is this: egregious violations of values require public stands. Behind-the-door consideration, though sometimes required for sound reasons, does not by itself meet the needs of the broader community. Leadership requires decision-making, and good decision-making requires the expression of core values.

If, for example, a widely known incident of racism is only privately addressed by a chair with the person who engaged in the racist behavior and not publicly addressed, then those who have heard about the incident conclude that nothing has been done and that the chair is complicit. Addressing the matter in private will never be enough, when the situation is one that requires a public stance and statement, such as an egregious violation of a core value.

In such a case, the chair could retain his or her role as moral leader if the chair had stated in a faculty meeting something to the effect that such behavior will not be condoned and that an apology had been asked for and given. Recall the case involving Dr. Special. There, the chair made a statement publicly that he had asked Dr. Special to apologize. It did not matter whether Dr. Special did so; what mattered was that the community knew the chair's stance on the values at stake.

As another example, a former graduate student comes forward to accuse her mentor of fudging his results. She does this fearing what it might mean for her career. You do what you can to protect her and begin your inquiry into scientific misconduct. In the end, a distinguished group of scientists conclude that the results have been fabricated. In this case, both the journals and NIH are notified of the findings. The retraction of the papers by the journal is public notice.

Gardner has suggested that values decay over time. Societies that keep their values alive do so not by escaping the process of decay but by processes that allow and encourage regeneration [2]. This is a fundamental aspect of the leader's responsibility to help the group survive.

References

1. Collins J. Good to great. New York: HarperCollins; 2001.
2. Gardner J. On leadership. New York: Free Press; 1990. p. 13–4.

Chapter 14
Stimulating Change Without Enduring a Coup

The ultimate test of a leader is whether he or she can fundamentally change the direction and strategy of an organization. Managers can make the trains run on time, but the leader can change where they are going and how they get there. There is nothing more rewarding and exhilarating than enabling organizational change and, with the benefit of hindsight and history, achieving subsequent validation that the collective interests of the organization have been served.

Leading large-scale change requires just about every bit of information in this book and every skill we've attempted to identify and explain.

- The leader has to be trusted and viewed as having the best interests of the group at heart. Trust is the basis for real leadership.
- The leader has to be able to navigate through the formal and informal organizations and know when to focus on which part. The key is to align both the formal and informal organizations so they work in a complementary fashion. Unfortunately, a frequent approach to change involves using the *power* of formal organizational mechanisms while disregarding the *authority and influence* of the informal organization.
- The leader has to understand and leverage the culture, values, and archetypes, including historically based images and symbols, and use them to move forward.
- The leader has to accept that authority must be earned and bestowed on him or her. Hierarchal, title-based power is limited in academic institutions.
- The leader has to be able to formulate a relatively simple message and be willing to repeat it.
- The leader needs to show perseverance, stamina, and courage to withstand criticism.
- And the leader needs to mediate conflict, understand interests, and find solutions benefitting everybody when they are there and stand by when there is an evident lack of consensus or agreement.

© Springer International Publishing Switzerland 2015
J.L. Houpt et al., *Learning to Lead in the Academic Medical Center*,
DOI 10.1007/978-3-319-21260-9_14

Armed with these ideas in mind, we suggest two additional ideas. They are based on a single observation that academics overvalue ideas. We assume that a good idea will sell itself. The attitude too often is to announce an idea and believe that it will attract followers. But that approach doesn't work—committee reports, for example, collect dust.

Identify All the Players Who Might Have a Stake in the Change Agenda

We recommend a strategy that involves up to seven sets of players. The players are the following: (1) you, whether a dean, chair, center director, or division head; (2) your boss; (3) the mafia (these are people who can influence events with a phone call and are sometimes outside your ability to influence—donors, alumni, trustees, legislators, former presidents, editors, the newspaper, and so forth—these people are much more often part of playing field for deans than chairs, because they are part of the dean's constituency, but they can affect chairs as well); (4) your staff and leadership team, including the formal organization; (5) the faculty; (6) the village elders; and (7) the AMC or university attorney and the HR department.

In initiating a change agenda, you need to think about each of these seven sets of players, understand their role, and develop a plan for them to help you accomplish your objectives. The plan needs to be framed in terms of their interests or shared interests. You don't need all of the sets of players for every change agenda, but you will need some for every agenda. For example, the addition of a biologic component to the psychiatry department requires a plan of action involving only the faculty. If there had been resistance involving a group of faculty going to the dean, then the field enlarges to include the dean; if a disgruntled faculty member treated an influential person in the community and goes to him or her to complain, then you need a plan for that person (probably one involving the mafia).

Likewise, if someone goes to the press, then you need to involve your communication people. The strategy is to take on the agenda with as few players as possible but to anticipate a larger set and act accordingly. The ability to anticipate the presence and actions of these various characters is imperative to a successful change strategy.

Imagine these two scenarios. In one, the CEO of the health system is buying a hospital in order to consolidate services and improve patient care, and there is no internal or external reaction. It's seen as business as usual. In this case, the CEO engages the board and his or her boss if there is one, the communication staff, and the attorney, perhaps a merger/acquisition law firm, and proceeds to do whatever is needed.

In a second scenario, a competing local hospital claims foul and calls a press conference, claiming predatory, monopolistic activity. The local television stations get involved, the legislature intervenes, the trustees get calls, the quiescent faculty become aroused and oppose the deal because they see it conflicting with the health system's mission, and pretty soon everyone has an opinion. In this case, a strategy needs to be developed that involves each set of players.

You can never be sure that you'll avoid a coup, but you have your best chance of doing so by addressing each set of actors. If you skip a set or can't get one on board, you will run into trouble. And be respectful; try to avoid surprising the players. This is especially true with your bosses. In our experience, the cardinal sin for the boss is to be surprised. Change requires a well-timed communication strategy.

The AMC or university attorney and the HR staff deserve special attention. Your relationship to them is important to your success. You want them to try to help you meet your objectives, rather than holding you back in an effort to protect the institution. Often it's tempting to do something and then ask forgiveness, but if that becomes your mode of operation, you will have a hard time getting these players on your side. You need to bring them in early. Try "I'd like to talk with you to see if there is a way that x can be done" rather than "I want to do this." The former question encourages them to think with you about whether something is possible, while the latter encourages a "yes" or "no." Over time they will determine if you are trustworthy and either help you or put brakes on you.

There Has to Be an Implementation Strategy

A good plan well executed will beat a great plan poorly executed every time. Another reason why so many committee reports collect dust is that committees rarely develop implementation plans for their often-valuable ideas. Committees frequently make recommendations, but never tell you how to get from here to there. And more often than not, the recommendations never get from here to there.

To devise an implementation strategy, you need to cultivate two different groups: the policy people, that is, those persons who will give you advice on how to move forward, and the change agents, those who will endure the insults and resistance but get the job done. To implement, you need to break down what you are trying to do into smaller bits—what needs to be done, who is responsible for doing it, and what time lines should be put into place, and the wonks and the change agents have different roles in this process.

AMCs have many talented policy thinkers. It's a role that most chairs, faculty, village elders, and even others outside the university relish. They are bright and they have the institution's best interests at heart. But they are not going to fight for your ideas or use their social capital to advance what they see as your cause. People up or down the line often step away, if their own interests have not benefitted and they aren't engaged independently.

Change agents, that is, people who will take an arrow for you, are less common. They may be among your chairs and village elders, but more likely are among your staff. These people see their job as doing your bidding. They also can be found among the people we have called the mafia. These are influential members of the community who believe in you and support you. Every really successful dean or vice president we've seen has had his or her own staff as well as external warriors.

You can usually look to the hospital to see this dynamic at work. Every success-ful hospital CEO we've encountered has had a loyal COO or CFO to carry out his or her will. They are the focal point of complaints, but they get the job done.

Once you find these change agents, you need to support them. People will com-plain about them and ask you to stop them or to get rid of them. But you need to support them, or no one will do the job for you.

> I've seen transitions in leadership where the new leader didn't wish to support these people because of their baggage and so they left or were forced out. Unless they were replaced with similar types, operations fell apart.

To summarize, we've taken our understanding of culture, the formal and infor-mal organization, the nature of authority, and the lessons from persuasion and added in two important features of organizational change—understanding the players and their interests and having an implementation plan. Becoming proficient at change that is grounded in these principles has helped us. We believe it will increase your chances of success.

Additional Points About Change

There are additional interesting points from the literature and our own experience in trying to initiate a change agenda.

1. People resist change even when it's a good idea.
No matter how good it looks on the surface, it will be resisted. Successful change requires acceptance of this phenomenon but the willingness to move forward any-way. You should never assume that change will be easy; it will always meet resistance.

> I used to be surprised by this and wonder why people didn't see that a potential change was actually in their best interest. However, I came to see that leading an organization to change requires a leader to deal with the most fundamental forces of human nature.
>
> First, as humans we seek our own self-interest, or, at least, what we think is in our best interest. Organizational change is seen as disrupting the status quo and throwing into ques-tion whether we will be winners or losers. I learned that in the imagination of those affected by change, a universe of potential poor outcomes has been created, including the sinister "what-if" option. If you can identify this erosive fear and address it, you can make your job easier. That's why talking to people before you more forward with change is so important. Again, the listening skills of the leader are all important.
>
> Second, as human beings we crave stability and a sense of permanence, and we make our choices accordingly. We choose to work in those specialties that seem to fit our sensi-bilities, skills, and preferences. We select AMCs as places to work because we feel some kindred spirit even if we can't always pinpoint what it is. We feel comfortable there.

Finding and operating in our comfort zones are so appealing that we resist change even if is not in our best interest. We stay in dysfunctional relationships or stay with dead-end jobs. Organizations can suffer from the same dynamics, i.e., choices can be made that impair their ability to function in healthy, adaptive ways.

Even successful practices from the past can become dysfunctional and maladaptive-organizational ossification is a function of our need for security and predictability. This is one of the great challenges leaders in AMCs face when they have to address organizational inertia and resistance to change.

And finally, sometimes the proposed change requires sacrifice; it hurts us but is good for the organization. This topic is addressed in Chap. 6 on The Importance of Emotional Intelligence where we indicated the need for the transformational leader to move faculty and staff from a position of what's good for me to a position of what's good for us. Maybe resistance to change is best summarized in the adage that the devil you know is better than the devil you don't know. All of these reasons make initiating change very tough. You often need a push or a threat.

2. Most change is stimulated in response to a theat.

It's useful to distinguish between change that is forced on you and is purely reactive or catch-up and change that is made in anticipation of something happening in the future. The literature suggests that organizations operate in three different change modes. These tendencies were described in a now classic Club of Rome study (commissioned by the wealthy membership—people who own international businesses), which identified three kinds of leadership/learning [1].

The primary one is maintenance learning, which creates a reactive mode of operating where everyone is simply trying to keep up. If the world changes faster than the organization, then everyone ends up in a shock learning mode, playing a desperate game of catch-up, often with diminishing resources. The third alternative they describe is anticipatory learning where you change before you have to. This is a major leadership challenge—it is very rare—but when a leader is able to create the proper forums, alliances and actions, anticipatory learning can happen and an organization can deal with the challenges of the future by creating responses to meet the threats.

The Rothschilds are often cited as an example of anticipatory learning—they were arguably the first financial organization to recognize the value of speed of information and thus used carrier pigeons in the nineteenth century to relay information between the capital markets of Europe to outperform their rivals [2]. Unfortunately few organizations operate by anticipating the need for change and by driving it from within.

Sometimes in AMCs we operate in the maintenance mode or shock mode because of things that are imposed on us without much warning. The largest recently have been financial: the balanced budget act of the late 1990s, the Affordable Care Act, the rate adjustments to Medicare, some states' decisions not to expand Medicaid, the frequent declines in NIH funding, decreasing state support for higher education, etc. If those jolts aren't enough, we face mandates requiring change from our accrediting bodies: the LCME, the ACGME, and the Joint Commission, to name just some.

Our observation is that AMCs do relatively well in responding to these kinds of immediate threats, where we function in a maintenance mode and avoid the shock mode. This isn't different from most other organizations. Immediate external threats require relatively quick executive action. It's obvious to the faculty and while they may complain, they don't start coups over such actions. They view the organization and its leader as victims who were dealt a bad hand and had to play it. The enemy is external.

AMCs do a much less effective job at anticipatory change. Anticipatory change differs from maintenance or shock mode because the consequences of the threats that impel anticipatory change are less obvious, often debatable, and consequently require faculty buy-in and input. Such change takes longer, requires more energy, and is sometimes just avoided. Health system network development and hospital consolidation were born out of perceived external financial threats and were fashioned in anticipatory mode.

Some AMCs still have not addressed these threats. On the other hand, the responses of some AMCs to these threats have been very successful, though some have led to large financial losses. The point is that anticipatory change necessarily invites subsequent evaluation. With this kind of change, the leader is subject to review and scrutiny at a level that doesn't occur with maintenance or shock mode interventions. Such changes are seen as responses to the outside, something we had to do, whereas anticipatory changes are seen as more voluntary and open to greater criticism.

Thus, an irony exists. You want a CEO to act in an anticipatory mode. But a CEO who acts in an anticipatory mode opens himself or herself up to criticism, whereas the CEO who operates in a maintenance mode avoids criticism. Unfortunately, the board often does not know the industry well enough and thinks the second CEO who is actually avoiding anticipatory actions is doing well because his or her actions don't draw scrutiny. Only ten years hence do they realize it, and then it is often too late. However, anticipatory changes can be transformative.

3. A crisis is not to be avoided; it is an opportunity to be embraced.

Because most change is stimulated from external forces, crisis is your best friend. Inexperienced leaders bemoan crises and usually frighten the faculty with their doomsday scenarios, robbing them of hope. Seasoned leaders look on crises as opportunities. Rahm Emanuel grabbed national headlines when he said, "You never want a crisis to go to waste: it's an opportunity to do important things that you would otherwise avoid"[3]. Harvard University political philosopher Michael Sandal said "taking office at a time of crisis doesn't guarantee greatness, but it can be an occasion for it"[4].

The lesson to be learned is that the greater the crisis, the greater the opportunity for transformative change. Earlier in the book we spoke of biography and concluded that history's verdict has been that greatness is assigned when the man or woman meets the situation and does something transformative with it.

One of my health system board chairs said it slightly differently; "great institutions always seem to come up with the right leader at a time of crisis, whereas mediocre ones simply do not."

Some people are stimulated by crisis and others are burdened by it. Imagine these two scenarios. *You're the dean at a state medical school, and the legislature has cut the budget by 10 %. This occurs after a few years of smaller cuts or no raises, and the easy things have already been done. Dean #1 says we're going to stop our current searches and put in 10 % across-the-board cuts.* "I feel really bad but there is nothing more we can do until the legislature turns things around." *The chairs feel defeated.*

Dean #2 approaches it differently, indicating "as you've heard, we have to absorb a 10 % cut. This means we need to cut back. But we need to cut back so that when we come out of this recession, we are stronger, not weaker. That means we will need to be smaller, but I emphasize we must and can be stronger. It's like pruning a tree. It gets smaller in the present but it grows bigger and stronger in the end."

"I'm going to begin the process by appointing a committee of faculty and chairs to look at the dean's office budget and it will tell us what services are not needed and what are. Their goal is not to cut 10 % across-the-board. That just makes everybody weaker. Their job is to cut 10–15 % if possible from programs of questionable utility. And if we can cut more than 10 %, we'll have money to invest as we cut back. If not, we'll stop at the 10 % mark. Then we'll set up a process for all of you to do the same with your departments."

We believe there are three roles a leader must play in managing crises with setbacks and adversity. First, consistent with the view that leaders define reality for their followers, the leader (dean #2 in the case above) *frames the reality,* e.g., "we have to deal with an adversity that we need to use as an opportunity to become stronger." The keyword that frames this situation and provides an interpretive framework for everyone is *opportunity.*

Second, the leader must elaborate and *tell a simple but compelling story* that, like all stories, has a beginning, middle, and end. "Here is what we have to deal with, here is what we are going to do, and here is the outcome (we are stronger)." The tone of the story is as important as the content. The confidence and positive belief of the boss is one of the most powerful predictors of employee performance—this is most certainly true for the boss who is also a leader.

Third, the leader has to *define specific ways for people to become involved* in dealing with the crisis and then commit to these ways personally. "I go first, but you follow. You'll be involved all along the way."

As Gary Hamel, a noted strategist, observes, "People tend to operate in one of two ways in a turbulent environment of rapid change—either as a victim or an activist. Involving them allows them to move from the role of passive/reactive victim to one of proactive activist" [5]. Such direct, hands-on involvement lowers their levels of stress and enhances their effectiveness. As the dean #2 communicated, "We're all in this together. This is an opportunity. We'll consult with HR and the AMC lawyer to do it the right way, but I'm convinced we can do it."

The Base Level of Stress Within an Organization Dictates Strategy

One of the most powerful models for understanding the role that leaders must play during a time of rapid change and high stress is the classic Yerkes–Dodson Law [6]. Based originally on animal research, the model has been extended and developed with continued research on human subjects in a variety of settings. Simply put, stress can be a motivator of effective performance *up to a point*, beyond which performance declines based on the deleterious effects of stress. With this perspective the leader should assume one of three broadly defined roles, based on the ambient stress.

In those organizations where both performance and stress are relatively low, the leader's job is to inspire, energize, and drive performance upward. One could argue that 90 % of the literature on leadership addresses this area of performance—leading the charge into a desired future using every possible means. These are often traditional, stable, and comfortable seniority-based organizations. They are precedent driven with low levels of employee motivation and engagement. Leaders often have to make a dramatic entrance to gain people's attention and elevate their commitment and mobilize high levels of performance.

In contrast, some environments are high stress and high anxiety, and people are, at the extreme, protecting their jobs rather than doing their jobs. In part this is a function of being overstressed so that their adaptive responses and intelligence are compromised by stress-based stereotypical flight-or-fight responses. In this kind of environment, the leader needs to get actively involved in encouraging, coaching, counseling, informing, and supporting his or her people. The necessary roles and skills of the leader can be very different. As one IBM executive wryly observed, "Oh I get it. In one case the leader is comforting the afflicted, and in the other the leader is afflicting the comfortable."

In the middle zone—the sweet spot for optimal organizational performance—the leader is attuned to his or her people and able to *both* inspire and motivate while *also* informing, coaching, and encouraging based on what specific individuals and groups need. This kind of leadership requires the leader to be capable of titrating and balancing the levels of challenge and support that are required to sustain optimal performance. Such leadership requires the highest levels of personal commitment and awareness to respond to the ongoing needs of others.

Pay Attention to Timing and to Getting the Right People on Board

Change requires a strategy that anticipates the proper timing and identifies the best people who are capable of carrying it out.

As we indicated earlier, some issues are low-hanging fruit and some are third rail issues. You must know the difference. Low-hanging fruit represents potential changes that benefit everyone and are in keeping with existing values, like adding a research core that is funded by a donor. These changes are usually easily accomplished and can be carried out at any time, including in your first few months.

Third rail issues are issues that reach deep into the culture of an organization and appear to threaten core values. One example would be changing the compensation plan or changing tenure. These changes should never be attempted until you are well into your term, have earned your authority, and have deeply involved all who are affected.

Sometimes you just have to wait until you "get the right people on the bus"—a phrase popularized by Collins in *Good to Great* [7]. Simply stated, you can't ask people to do what they are incapable of doing. If you are a dean with a chair who just can't get done what you need to be done, for whatever reason, you need to wait until you get a new chair. Another way of saying this is that change requires patience, timing, and the right people. Think of it as a multi-act play. Many lack patience and so fail in efforts to stimulate change.

The ultimate test of a leader's credibility and effectiveness can be measured by the willingness of others to follow him or her into a change agenda. Whether the individual can carry out the agenda will determine how he or she is judged. To carry out change, the leader needs to master the skill sets we have attempted to describe in this book. It also requires the leader to develop these skills in others. The effect of the latter is to nurture leadership for the organization's future, which may be among the highest skills of a leader.

References

1. Meadows D, Randas J, Behrens W. Limits to growth. NY: Signet; 1971.
2. Ferguson N. The richest dynasty in history? The house of Rothschild. NY: Viking; 1998.
3. Emanuel R. NY Times, November 7, 2008. p. 19.
4. Sandal M. NY Times, November 5, 2008. p. 31.
5. Hamel G, Prahalad PK. Competing for the future. Boston: Harvard Business School Press; 1994.
6. Yerkes RM, Dodson JD. The relation of strength of stimulus to rapidity of habit-formation. J Comp Neurol Psychol. 1908;18:459–82.
7. Collins J. Good to great. New York: HarperCollins; 2001.

Chapter 15
A Final Word to Applicants and Search Committees: Picking the Right People for Leadership Roles the First Time

Having read this book, we hope you are convinced that people can learn to become better leaders. But it is probably also clear that recruiting the right leaders in the first place saves you much time and effort. Getting the right people has spawned a huge industry. Corporate America spends huge amounts developing their talent and choosing who they believe their next leaders should be. AMCs recognize this, and search firms are now commonplace for higher positions. Leadership development programs have been created and implemented in many AMCs. However, some of our programs are not fully developed and fall short of corporate programs.

We have suggested earlier in Chap. 9 on Recruitment: Negotiation in Action that we believe that there are three aspects to successfully picking the right person. We suggest first that you use an issue-oriented approach to recruitment. Carried out correctly, that approach provides the most information about how candidates set priorities, their capacity to assess strengths and weaknesses, their valence toward the existing faculty, and their ability to assess culture and to formulate strategy. In that chapter, we also noted that successful recruitment requires a fit of the candidate and the position and, in the cases of leadership positions, requires an additional set of "soft skills" based on emotional competencies.

This chapter builds on those latter two aspects: fit and emotional competencies. It considers the concept of fit from the point of view of the candidate. And it deals with the softer skills required in a leadership position from the point of view of the search committee.

By "soft skills" we mean those competencies required to lead a large organization: bringing people together, motivating, mediating conflict, stimulating change, and the others detailed in this book—that is, those that are based more in emotional competencies than in technical or cognitive realms.

In short, this chapter speaks to the applicant and how he or she might decide to take on a leadership role and to search committees and how they might pick the right candidate. Picking the right person sounds simple, but it is not. Everyone who reads this book can point to poor choices, as we can.

© Springer International Publishing Switzerland 2015
J.L. Houpt et al., *Learning to Lead in the Academic Medical Center*,
DOI 10.1007/978-3-319-21260-9_15

And perhaps that is the correct starting point. Picking people is an imprecise science. We do a pretty good job of picking faculty members, but we are not so good in picking from among them those who should take on leadership roles. So that's where we will start—why it's so hard to pick the right leadership candidate. We'll then move to what aspiring applicants should consider and finish with some final thoughts for search committees.

Why It's So Hard to Pick the Right Candidate

We think the biggest obstacle to picking the right candidate is that the skills that will be required haven't been demonstrated yet. Whether you are an internal or external candidate, you are moving to a bigger stage and haven't had the opportunity to develop the skills that will be required there. It's always a guess whether the person will develop into the job. Can the good faculty member become a good division head; can the division head become a good chair; or can the chair become a dean? Can he or she deal with the increasing scope, complexity, and ambiguity and make the transition from an individual contributor to a team member and/or team leader? These questions point to just a few of an impressive, sometimes daunting list of developmental steps you'll need to conquer, which we've enumerated in Appendix A. We've listed 18. If you read through them, we believe you will agree with us that they represent several potential pitfalls.

Second, in addition to being unable to anticipate a successful outcome to these developmental steps, you also can't predict that the skills already shown within one environment will translate to a new one. What works in one culture just might not work in a different one. There have been several rough transitions from NIH leadership roles to running AMCs and vice versa, from academia to the government sector, from the pharmaceutical industry to academia, and also from one AMC to another—e.g., a Darwinian institution to a care and feeding institution.

You also can't predict whether personality traits that may have been minimally detrimental in one milieu will or won't become big problems in a different setting. We've mentioned this earlier, but perfectionism in a successful lab director may work in that one setting, but not on a larger stage. In a smaller setting, you might get away without delegating and by micromanaging, but not so in a larger, more complex environment.

In summary, there are a lot of things you just can't know: whether a person will successfully master the developmental steps outlined in Appendix A; whether what works in one setting will survive the cultural transition to another place; and finally, whether relatively harmless personality traits in one setting will be magnified in a larger setting. We thus ought to begin this process of selecting applicants appropriately humbled. We suggest some things that might mitigate potential failures. First, we consider what aspiring candidates should be considering about themselves, and then we examine the processes and procedures of search committees to improve our odds in picking the right candidate.

A Word to Aspiring Applicants

We'd advise potential applicants for these jobs to consider four questions before committing to a leadership position. (1) Why would I want this job *now* and does it fit my maturational curve? (2) What does the job entail and do I want to do it? (3) Is this job a "fit" for me? (4) Are the resources available to do the job?

Why Would I Want This Job Now?

The "right" answer is that "I can make a greater contribution by taking a leadership position than by continuing to do my individual work"—whether it is teaching, research, or patient care. But while this answer may be the correct one, candidates often do not consider it. Success in the AMC is marked by the acquisition of resources and status. We live in a competitive culture in the AMC where seeking out recognition and resources is automatic. Taking a leadership position provides both. Such positions offer more money and more hard-money salary support, and they certainly provide status and recognition. People find themselves, as Steve Wartman suggests in the Foreward, as "accidental leaders."

A better motivation than resources and status is the judgment that you can make a contribution by helping others develop their careers. This means acknowledging that what you do individually-your research, teaching, or patient care—will have less impact than what you can achieve if you can enable and encourage a much larger group to work in a way that collectively makes a greater contribution. The amount of individual orientation you need to give up increases as you move up the administrative level. Division heads are expected to keep and, in fact, lead in their research or patient care; chairs are expected to continue some academic pursuits; whereas deans to a large degree focus on the managerial and leadership aspects of their positions. As we noted in Chaps. 4–6, this other orientation involves moving psychologically to a point where you can experience pleasure from others doing well rather than just from your own individual work. This movement is part of your maturational curve. The first maturational task of adulthood according to Ericson is to focus and succeed at a job, and, in the AMC, you do that by gaining resources and recognition [1]. A later maturational task is to enter into a mentoring stage where others' success becomes paramount.

A second way to look at this question of maturation and life cycle is simply to focus on your chronological age. From your current age, imagine where you'll be at various points in the future. Assume a 10-year term (two five-year cycles) in a leadership position, and ask yourself what you would do at the end of it. For example, if you were in your late 40s and looking at a dean's position, the question would be what you might do in your late 50s. There are no "correct" ages to ask these questions and no right answers here. It only matters that you are beginning to put the questions into a life cycle perspective.

Having promoted the concept of maturational curve, we now have to add a caveat. The perfect job doesn't always come along at the perfect time. Sometimes you have to take things out of order. You just have to decide to take that leap or not.

If you get a leadership job early in your career (not your last job), keep some clinical or research skills. We often become "deskilled" in two years if we don't keep up or even sooner for certain specialties.

What Does the Job Entail and Do I Want to Do It?

We've been amazed at times that some in leadership positions don't understand what their job is. They see it as a narrow extension of what they've done before along with a dose of celebrity. They miss their responsibility to the collective whole and its welfare. We've seen chairs who view the job as enhancing their own area of research, or their own clinical area. We've seen chairs who believe their job is to keep their research going and to travel around the country becoming a celebrity. We've seen deans who view their job as meeting the ceremonial and celebrity aspects, but not the management aspects, or the opposite, where they are pleased to manage but abhor and avoid the ceremonial aspects.

Once you understand that it's not about your programs but about building the department's and others' success, you can review the skills outlined in this book— negotiating, conflict resolution, and change strategies—and assess where you are and decide if you've got the right set of skills for what's needed.

Is This Job a "Fit" for Me?

In Chap. 4 on Personality Traits and Leadership, we considered biographical approaches to understanding leadership and suggested that the "fit" is paramount to success. Admittedly, that judgment is easier made after the fact than before. Going forward, it is really hard, but here are a few personal anecdotal examples.

> When I was first looking at chair positions I was looking at Emory and one other program. At Emory, I saw a very complicated organizational format as it had clinical, teaching, and research programs at five different hospitals with different governance structures. The other program I was considering had one university owned hospital with the same governance structure as the medical school. The complexity at Emory was intriguing to me because I happen to feel comfortable with complicated social systems, and I thought I could make a greater contribution there because of that. Another person with a different set of interests and strengths would have been right to make a different choice.
>
> When looking at dean positions, I was attracted to UNC because I felt its values were similar to mine. I became impressed in my interviews with its sense of collegiality and its commitment to serve the people of the State. Having been a dean already, and knowing the pressures brought to bear by finances and rankings, I enjoyed the idea that there would be other existing values to be brought into play. Not that UNC lacked financial or ranking concerns, but they had other values that required some counter balancing. Others may have

been put off by competing values, and have found focusing on finances and rankings enough of a problem, but I liked the moral rudder that UNC had, and the added complexity did not bother me.

   At another time, I looked at a dean's position and concluded that the faculty had no interest in being "made over" as their administration was hoping for. It looked impossible to me, so I withdrew.

From these examples, we can make a few tentative suggestions. The Emory example suggests matching your interests/skills with what the job requires. The UNC example suggests that finding a match of values is as important as what the job requires. The final example suggests that it's important to find a job that is doable.

Thus, we have a short list for determining the "fit" in terms of matching skills with the job and personal values with institutional ones and an assessment of whether or not the job is doable. We're sure there are more points to consider as well.

With regard to values, we'd suggest reviewing Chap. 2 on Culture Is King and, specifically, the dichotomous values listed there. Decide which of those values exist in the AMC where you are thinking of going, and then see if those are your values. If you and the school have the same values, then you have a fit. If the values don't match, beware. More than likely, if you set out on a change agenda, you will run into conflict over the change because of the value difference, which will make your job more difficult.

In my experience coaching, many of the difficulties for which people were referred involved issues of "fit," and some mixture of culture and personality. The most common "misfits" were these. First, perfectionistic, judgmental people committed to excellence who were recruited to places where collegiality and getting along were the prevailing values, and where there was satisfaction with the status quo. Second, "executive" leaders in a "process" school or "Darwinians" in a "care and feeding" school resulted in the newly minted leader exercising his or her values in ways that made the faculty feel unimportant and inferior.

What Resources Are Necessary to Do the Job?

Understanding how to identify the resources necessary to do the job is addressed in Chap. 9, Recruitment: Negotiation in Action.

A Word to Search Committees

Search committees are the preferred method of choosing regular faculty and faculty in leadership positions. The higher the leadership post, the more formal and cumbersome the process becomes, and as a result, the more likely that process will find the wrong candidate. Hence, we think there is a need to look at the process: the composition of the search committee, its charge, and its method of interviewing. We've already argued that for higher leadership positions, behavioral and emotional skills account for much of the success. The candidates' intellect, as shown in publications and other academic credentials, has to be at a level to command respect. Without an acceptable level of intellect as shown in their scholarship, they will have a hard time getting authority bestowed on them by the faculty. But on top of that, they need evidence of performance.

> Behaviorally, they should have a track record of success in building programs. In my mind, the best accolade I can hear is that this person left every place he or she was better than he or she found it. I prefer multiple, sometimes smaller successes to single large dramatic successes. The reason is that often the real work was done by someone other than the person taking credit, and luck and timing are part of every success. But multiple successes bespeak a pattern of extracting the best out of every circumstance, taking advantage of timing, and finding your luck.

The third set of skills are emotional ones, and this is where most search committees have trouble. We've traced some of those reasons already, so we'll now focus on what we can do to maximize our ability find those with emotional intelligence.

Find Someone Who Avoids Glib "Business Speak"

Picking a leader begins with an understanding of the multiple missions of the AMC—education, research, and patient care—and the leader's fundamental role of representing the interests of everyone within the group.

The leader must understand that the missions are in conflict at times and that he or she needs to balance them. The needs of the hospital can overwhelm the normal architecture of a premiere department. For example, if you are in a research-intensive AMC, the department of medicine should likely lead the way in grant activity. Financial incentives focused only on clinical productivity would cripple the research mission and thus lower the school's and university's and/or AMC's rank. In another example, if your emergency room is filled with psychiatry patients, the psychiatry department can't shift all of its residents to the emergency room instead of other rotations without jeopardizing their residency competitiveness and accreditation. From the hospital's perspective, the medical school and its departments can't view the hospitals as a bank and not respond to its needs. The AMC needs to mount a comprehensive and competitive clinical program in order to be successful. For example, if you need five more anesthesiologists to meet surgical needs, you have to find a way to provide them.

Simple as this may sound, it is not. Find someone who understands the complexity beyond the jargon. What you too often hear is that we need to "align incentives" or "reward productivity." This sounds good and often appeals to business leaders if they are on the search committee, because it does work in their world. It works where there are accepted single endpoints, but not with multiple, conflicting endpoints. But it does not work for those clinical departments with a substantial NIH research portfolio, like medicine, pediatrics, psychiatry, or neurology, for example. Increased volumes can detract from the research mission, as can incentivizing only for clinical productivity. In some departments, increasing clinical volumes may actually decrease the bottom line. Different departments need to be incentivized differently.

While clinical care has its ally in increased revenue, and research has its ally in increased discovery, more research, and heightened status, there is no natural constituency group for medical education. Education just needs to be doggedly supported from above and actively supported. Obviously, over time organizations can theoretically incent for all missions. And that's good. What needs to be avoided is the idea that one size fits all.

> The caution about "glib" candidates leads to one final thought on this subject. I become terribly suspect of a candidate who says nothing unpredictable in an interview. If I leave an interview and I hear nothing that causes me to look at an issue differently, or at least offers a contrasting perspective, I become concerned. Creativity and the ability to look at a situation from various perspectives is hard to measure, and the CV is certainly not perfect in that regard. Membership in learned societies also does not measure these qualities. But you might get a glimpse of them in the interview. I want to leave an interview saying to myself, "I learned something new there; I hadn't looked at it that way before."

Eliminate the Personality Disorders

Collins [2] concludes that boards of directors often make the mistake of choosing someone from the outside who is "larger than life." And as a general rule, larger-than-life people are narcissistic, as a generous dose of narcissism is often required to be "larger than life." In Collins' study, the level 5 leader came from within in a vast number of cases, and external potential level 5 leaders were passed over because they didn't excite or entertain the search committee in the interview.

We covered much of this in Chap. 5 on Managing Personality Disorders in the Workplace and some in Chap. 9 on Recruitment: Negotiation in Action. Listen to the candidate to see if he or she shares credit with others or takes all the credit personally. If you find yourself totally enraptured by someone, ask yourself if this person is real. If after a while you start wondering if all of what you're hearing could be true, then pay attention to your feelings.

> I was sitting next to a successful businessman at a UNC dinner event a while ago. He had just chaired the search for a person high in the administrative ranks at UNC. He had hired many people in his lifetime, and so the topic of conversation shifted to this book and our common interest in how you pick the right person. His comment was, "I listen to hear if they talk in 'I's' or 'we's'. If I hear too many 'I's', I get nervous and immediately call where they've been and make sure they aren't too self-centered."

Do Your Homework

CVs contain a lot of information about a candidate's academic credentials and accomplishments, but almost nothing about their EI. You shouldn't rely only on the interview or even on search firms. You must make calls to find out about the candidate yourself.

But you must also find sources that will tell you the truth. The truth is always out there. You just have to find it. Calling strangers cold will often not give you the truth. And calling the dean or chair of the department, while it is the courteous thing to do, will not necessarily give you the truth. People just don't want to get into the messy stuff of relating someone's faults to a stranger.

As we mentioned in Chap. 9 on Recruitment: Negotiation in Action, the surest way to find the truth is to call a person who is a friend of yours in the institution where the potential recruit is now. Only people with allegiance to you will tell the truth. If they are not in the same department, call them anyway, because even if they do not know the person, they have a network of friends who will give them the true story.

Using Search Firms

Search firms can enhance a search, but if you outsource the entire search to them, you could be disappointed. We believe that search firms can add value, particularly in the searches for higher-level positions—deans and above and some chairs.

Firms bring knowledge of the market—the current level of recruitment packages, the positions open at this time, the current difficulty in closing searches in that area, and most valuably a list of people currently looking at these jobs. Search firms bring their own lists, which sometimes include all the people they considered in their last search who didn't get offered or who didn't take the job. They will supplement the list you create through your ads and personal solicitations. Search firms can also vet candidates on a preliminary basis.

They offer many advantages, but they can be a detriment as well. You have to understand how they make their money and how they get their information. They often get paid a set amount based on a percentage of the yearly compensation of the person selected. This incents them to suggest that you pay top dollar and to finish the search quickly. They get paid when you pick someone, so they want you to be excited about the pool. If you are excited and if you miss the first candidate, they want you to move on to the second "because the pool is so good," rather than asking the firm to start over.

Finally, be a little suspicious of the vetting of the candidate that the search firm does. They meet the candidates and get many who might not want to jump into a public search because they are not ready to reveal their candidacy to their home institution. This is a great help because these are often top-flight people to whom you would never get access if you did the search without the firm. But the downside to this confidentiality is that the firm may agree to only ask referees that the potential candidate approves. This almost always excludes the boss and others with important perspectives. So the candidate gives the names of close confidantes and mentors whom they can trust to say the right things. As you might guess, the candidate's controlling the access to referees produces a glowing dossier. It is about the worst way to find out a candidate's weaknesses. Thus, you have to do your own vetting and do your own homework. You also have to independently determine compensation.

Work on Your Interview Technique

It is essential for you to have an idea of the kinds of thing you want to learn in an interview.

Here is a potential list I've found useful. Is the recruit self-centered or other centered? Does the recruit have a track record of improving the program every place he or she has been? Is the person someone who wins the loyalty of others? Does he or she have colleagues who want to follow him or her to the next place? Has the person taken a stand for the interests of the institution? Is the person someone who gives others credit?

In the interview you look for these characteristics, but how you ask questions is critical. You need to ask open-ended questions first and then clarify with more close-ended ones. An open-ended question does not give away the answer, and thus gives you more useful information. For example, I'd ask a chair candidate for a research-intensive department, "What would you like to do with this department?" If the individual begins talking about how the existing department could add to his or her own research program and how the department could be a leader in his or her area, then you don't have a level 5 leader. You may decide to take him or her strategically because your goal is to recruit that individual to your school and use the department as bait. But rest assured, you've just recruited a glorified lab director. If, on the other hand, he or she says "I think that the young people show a lot of promise," or "I think a recruit in this area could improve this area of research," or "We might want a more senior member here because we need to mentor the younger investigators," or "I see a lot of potential for joint programs with other departments," then you have someone who understands that the job is to build the department, not just the person's own research program.

If this nondirective approach is not working, then another line of questioning worth pursuing is to ask the person for an experience where he/she tried to help someone else succeed and how it worked out. You can judge their enthusiasm for this type of work by the amount of passion and interest they show in answering the question. If they report that they tried but failed, then you can not only judge their interest in mentoring, but you have learned not that they failed but that they can acknowledge mistakes and learn from them.

Pick the Search Committee the "Right" Way

The way we pick our committees is based on sound principles but has negative, unintended consequences. It also sets the stage for them to interview the wrong way. We look for members who broadly represent the AMC and/or the university. This sounds like such a good idea. The candidate needs to work with a broad group of people and pull groups together. We're committed to processes that are open to all constituents, where all feel they have a voice. But you need to address the consequences of this approach.

Here is what happens. Say we're looking for a dean. We pick a scientist and a clinician, and then we add a staff member, an alum, and then a student and maybe resident, then a fixed-term faculty member, and then a business person or trustee or community representative. We address the demographics.

The committee meets and the members look around. The basic scientist realizes that she "represents" the basic scientists, the fixed-term individual figures that he "represents" the fixed termers, the staff member that she represents the staff, and so on. The committee members come to believe that they are there to represent the interest of their constituency or "union." Even if they are slow to get it, by the time they meet, some basic scientists have taken the basic scientist committee member aside and said, "You're the only one there who knows science—you need to protect us." And so it goes throughout the committee.

Thus, the committee members behave as if their job is to protect their sector (remember the leader's first task). Rather than searching for a leader who can bridge or balance competing interests and inspire, the committee members look and argue for the person who best represents their constituents. Further, the idea of picking people who have experience picking people and maybe have had some success in doing so is usually not considered. The basic scientist in is the National Academy and may have had no substantial management responsibility. The student or house staff member may have been elected to a student or trainee office. But whether they have selected leaders and whether they have done it well is almost never considered.

We're not suggesting that we give up diverse, broadly representative groups—nor should we. But how about this simple suggestion? Look for people in all these categories who have shown that they can rise above parochial interest and look to the institution's interests. How about finding some people who have had to select people and how about some people who actually have done it well?

And how about a charge to the committee members along these lines?

> You were selected because you are respected and frankly because collectively you represent a broad representation of our institution. But you are not here to represent your constituency. You are here to represent the university and/or the AMC. Please, find a candidate who represents all the interests of the university, not just your sector. It's not about you and your interests; it's about the entire institution's interests.

> Unfortunately, this demographic approach to choosing the committee often spills over into how the interview is conducted. Usually the desire to have every interest represented also leads to large committees – at least 12 if not more. The committee may decide that everyone has to be asked the same set of questions, and that each member of the committee gets to ask a question. Everyone asks a question and then turns to the next person. There are almost no follow-up questions or efforts to clarify or probe particularly superficial answers. Almost always, the basic scientist is selected to ask the "research" question, the clinician the "clinical" question, and so forth, which only reinforces the silos. Further, the questions are almost always determined beforehand and are- "Give us your experience in developing... research programs,... clinical programs,... diversity, and so forth." There are no questions that ask the candidates to give their impressions of their visit, which would test their powers of observation and synthesis. As a psychiatrist, I can think of hardly any less useful ways to spend an interview session. This approach favors the glib, politically correct candidate who picks up on the unions in the room and like a good politician weaves in something for everybody.

> Here's how it should go. One member of the committee should lead off with a broad general question like "Share with us the impressions you formed on you visit." What the candidate says is important, but equally so is what he or she doesn't say. That opening leads to a second question, and then a third as you clarify both the candidate's interests and values. You can then turn to maybe 5 or 6 committee members who will ask specific questions,

and the rest can join in at the end to ask clarifying questions, or asking for things they didn't hear about.

You don't need to be a psychiatrist to be an effective search committee member. You do need to be experienced in interviewing, have a concern for your institution and not your own area only, and a history of making good selections. But the interview process needs to be changed to an open-ended format where you can ask follow-up questions.

Typical Interpersonal and Management Questions in Executive 360s

360s typically include cognitive and technical competences but also include questions on interpersonal and management style. The cognitive and technical competencies will be addressed in the CV and in your vetting of the candidate. In our experience, they are rarely the problem. The vulnerability is in assessing the interpersonal and management skills. We offer questions on interpersonal and management skills in Appendix B. We think it would be useful for committees to review these together before they do their background checks and interviews. It might be particularly useful to those on the committee with no managerial experience.

In conclusion, picking the right person is hard, but you can get better at it.

I've been thinking about this question of how to pick the right person for a long time. I know some people are really good at it and others are not. I can't tell you why. I've already offered up all the ideas I have on that. But as this chapter draws to a close and likewise this book, one thought and one image have come repeatedly to my mind. The psychiatrist in me wants to follow it.

When I was a psychiatry resident at Yale University a faculty member shared with me that the faculty was interested in whether they could predict who was going to be a good resident. So they ranked the residents into two categories: best and others. They then went back to the application folders and re-read them looking for any correlates. Only one jumped out. The final question on the interviewer's form was, "Did you like this person?" A yes correlated with the "best." You can find at least a few explanations. Maybe the people they liked at interview were the same people they liked later and so they were biased to call them the best. That is, maybe they weren't the best residents but just the best liked. Or maybe there is something in people who were liked that translated into their becoming better residents, more empathic, less arrogant, or something else.

As an aside, in my coaching I was always impressed with how much more latitude and allowance for errors were allowed for leaders who were liked, and how little the tolerance was for those who weren't liked.

I have this satisfying but recurring image. I'm retired from being dean. I am standing on the bridge that extends from the parking deck to the hospital and medical school. It is early morning because I'm going in for a rotator cuff repair. It's only 5:30 or 6:00 am, but the hospital is busy with energized people, purposely striding through the doors. They are fully engaged and when you look in their faces, you feel comforted as you approach your surgery.

At other times, the image is at night. I'm on the bridge again. I'm seeing all the research buildings with their lights ablaze. I'd learned as a dean that researchers are often night owls and I thought of them at work at night. The same feeling comes over me as I imagine them purposeful, energized, and committed to making this a better world through research.

And then I realize that I've had a career working with the brightest, most capable people in the world, and just maybe I made their life better and more productive. You recall where this book started – with the tremendous impact the AMC has, that is, the fact that it is the source of our medical workforce, the specialty units, the charity care, the Nobel prizes, the innovations in patient care, the basic research that will open up the discoveries of the future, and the fact of the sheer size of its economic impact.

Maybe picking the right person starts with a love of the mission, and seeing that the AMC is one of the most remarkable institutions in this country and in our history, and that we are privileged to be part of it. As an entity it surpasses anything we could do individually. Learning to deal with conflict and the personality disordered is a small price to pay for being a part of the bigger whole. All of us, when we stand on that bridge that overlooks both the medical school and its hospitals, find a sense of affection for and shared values with those who work there, and what makes us the "best" at our jobs is seen in an answer at the bottom of the interviewer's form, "I like them." Maybe the best of the leaders really want to work with those who work there, and want them to be the best they can be, and are prepared to deal with all the obstacles, because at some intra-psychic level they really like them and what they do. It's about them.

References

1. Ericson E. Childhood and society. W.W. Norton and Co.; 1950 (republished as a Penguin Book, 1969).
2. Collins J. Good to great. New York: HarperCollins; 2001.

Part IV
Cases for Discussion

Each of the chapters in this part consists of a case for group discussion. Each case presents a scenario designed to illustrate specific points and techniques discussed in Parts I–III. Each case concludes with an open-ended, single question, which in most of the cases is "What would you do?" The question is intended to encourage identification by the group of a wide variety of options and approaches. Our goal is to get as many opinions on the table as possible before we begin to narrow the discussion with more focused questions, which appear in Part V, Teaching Materials. We have found it valuable to encourage the early identification of different perspectives on what a particular case involves, especially for those who may initially miss the points that a case is designed to elicit. It is valuable for those individuals to think about what culture or beliefs or values or experiences produced their initial reactions and how they differed from those of others.

Chapter 16
Strategic Planning/Outside Consultants: Power and Authority, Vertical Hierarchies, and the Informal Organization

The university chancellor, with blessings from the Board of Trustees, initiated a comprehensive, two-year, university-wide strategic planning process that included the medical school. A large and prestigious national consulting firm was hired to help, and there followed a broad, open, 18-month process, out of which emerged a strategic plan with components for each school or college, including the medical school. Several members of the medical school faculty and the then dean of medicine served on key committees established as parts of the planning process that led up to the strategic plan itself.

Halfway through the planning process, the then dean developed serious health problems and resigned from his post, thus causing the chancellor to undertake a search for a new dean. Following a national search with participation from across the medical school, Dr. Rose, a well-known clinician/researcher and chair of the department of medicine at a prestigious New England Medical School, was hired with great anticipation. During his meetings with the search committee, the strategic plan was actively and supportively discussed. In Dr. Rose's negotiations with the chancellor, a key part of the chancellor's expectations and charge to him was to implement the medical school's portion of the strategic plan, which the chancellor and the trustees enthusiastically embraced, as did the new dean. A principal component of the plan involved the strategic acquisition of two well-located hospitals in the medical school's market area, as well as a number of clinical practices, so as to produce both a more integrated and more distributed system, better able to absorb the challenges associated with the redesign of the American healthcare system.

Since the plan was the product of broad input from faculty and staff across the university, was widely publicized, and was endorsed by the former dean, Dr. Rose immediately established an implementation committee to initiate the steps necessary to move forward with the plan's recommendations on hospital and practice acquisitions.

Immediately after the first steps were taken all hell breaks loose in the press, which characterizes the initiatives as "anticompetitive," "predatory," and "grasping."

© Springer International Publishing Switzerland 2015

J.L. Houpt et al., *Learning to Lead in the Academic Medical Center*,
DOI 10.1007/978-3-319-21260-9_16

The faculty expresses great consternation in the halls and clinics of the school and in faculty meetings, and it quickly becomes apparent to Dr. Rose that there is no internal or external consensus on the plan. Meanwhile, the chancellor and the trustees are expecting quarterly progress reports on implementation of the plan from the various deans, including the new medical school dean.

What would you do?

Chapter 17
Dr. Newby: Change, Getting Started, and Your Baby Is Ugly

You have just been named the chair of a clinical department at the Medical School of the People. You came from a prestigious private medical school. Your charge by the dean is to increase the research presence of the department and school.

Brimming with confidence, you are offered a reasonable package, but the state is going through a recession, state funding is decreasing, and third-party reimbursements are decreasing. Nevertheless, you start recruiting aggressively. Meanwhile, members of the department are talking in whispers about the wisdom of your pursuing these external recruitments when their compensation is threatened. A small chorus of faculty start saying out loud that maybe you ought to be using your package to bolster their income and not using it on outside people at least until things turn around economically.

Move forward a few weeks: two faculty come to see you to tell you that they are making plans to leave the department and to set up a practice in town, which of course will be in direct competition with the department. Also, these two people are the franchise, and if they leave, you will need to recruit new people to replace them.

You receive considerable counsel from the departmental faculty to retain these people but you have troubles from a number of points. They do not do research, and their field is one in which there are a pool of clinician/scientists.

So the area is high on your list as one in which you can meet the dean's charge to increase the research dollars. Even more disconcerting to you is that you do not consider the people you're asked to retain to be hard workers and in fact have concluded recently that you must put in a more incentive-laden compensation plan in order to get faculty working harder.

You permit the individuals to leave without any counter offer and form a committee to review the compensation plan. You charge the committee to look specifically at the department's incentives, and you provide them with a consulting firm to assist in getting national data as norms for work effort.

Move forward one year: three more faculty have left and your first two recruits have just joined your faculty. They are first rate and to get them you had to offer them more in salary than the existing faculty and give them the best space. You are

© Springer International Publishing Switzerland 2015
J.L. Houpt et al., *Learning to Lead in the Academic Medical Center*,
DOI 10.1007/978-3-319-21260-9_17

really pleased with them and have started three more searches. You are unaware of how these recruits are viewed. While you view them as great additions that everyone will welcome, they are instead seen by the existing faculty as evidence that you don't respect the existing people and the careers they have had.

Meanwhile, your committee on compensation is ready to report out and you receive a lackluster report that has something for every constituent but no real driving incentives and no robust benchmarks that you had hoped for. You talk to the committee chair, whom you handpicked, and he tells you that the committee was divided between those with a view like yours ("eat what you kill") and those concerned with tradition ("the plan needs to pay for teaching and citizenship and not just research and clinical work" which you interpret to mean "if we wanted to work that hard we'd have gone into private practice").

You get a call from the dean/CEO to tell you that he got a call from an important legislator who wanted to know "what is going on there." It appears that one of your department's faculty is the physician for this legislator, and he hears that you are driving away all the teachers in favor of researchers and bringing in all your own people from outside. The dean suggests that you need to show some interest in the old-timers. He makes it pretty clear that he wants everybody happy.

You leave the dean's office and wonder how you are going to handle this. Surely, if you side with the "eat what you kill group," it will get back to the legislator. If you confront the physician to the legislator, you could be charged with retaliation. If you don't put in the new compensation plan, you will never get the salaries up and your precious resources will be spent on the status quo. You have two really good recruits and potentially three on the line. If you get them, you are well on your way to having a transformed and terrific department. From your perspective, you are being asked to back off and support mediocrity, yet that is not what the dean told you when he hired you.

What would you do?

Chapter 18
Dr. Worksalot: Personality and Getting Started

Dr. Worksalot (Dr. W) was named chair of a clinical department one and one-half years ago. The dean selected him because his academic credentials were superior to anyone in the department, and the dean had fond hopes that Dr. W could add a much-needed NIH presence to the mostly clinical department. Early on, Dr. W. noted that the residents were not of a caliber acceptable to him, and, likewise, a couple of the faculty in his opinion should be released. He tried to energize the residency director to oust a resident at the year's end, but the residency director produced repeated evaluations showing that the resident did "acceptable" to more than "expected" work. The residency committee rejected the new chair's request.

Dr. W happened to be an introvert and perfectionist, as well a workaholic. This had been no problem in his meteoric rise as an academic because he could retreat to his lab and just work harder whenever stressed or when in jeopardy of losing his grant. This didn't bother his students and postdocs because they didn't expect much socializing or even basic social niceties. His reputation as borderline Asperger's didn't bother them either. They signed up despite that because they respected his IQ. Even though he was a taskmaster, it was no problem—his postdocs got jobs. It didn't matter that he never complimented them and needed endless data to make a decision. They didn't care because they preferred getting great training and a job to a warm and cuddly boss.

But the faculty didn't respond like his students. When the dean heard grumblings of dissatisfaction with Dr. W from the faculty, he hired a coach for him. The coach suggested that he "get out and around" and get to know people and show an interest in them instead of staying holed up in his office and sending out peremptory memos. Dr. W did as suggested. He reported the meetings a "great success." However, the faculty and residents who Dr. W visited felt as if they were "graded" on their responses to his inquiries and then found him lacking.

© Springer International Publishing Switzerland 2015
J.L. Houpt et al., *Learning to Lead in the Academic Medical Center*,
DOI 10.1007/978-3-319-21260-9_18

At the end of year one, he let an assistant professor go because he didn't believe the junior person was up to his standards. The person let go was a protégée of a much respected member of the department who had actually served one year as chief of the medical staff. Dr W doubted the value of the mentor as well.

By a year and a half, members of the faculty were grumbling about their new chair.

What would you advise Dr. Worksalot to do?

Chapter 19
Negotiating for a Center Director

You are chair of the department of cell biology. You are recruiting for a member of the department in proteomics. The successful candidate has to be not only an outstanding independent investigator but also the director of the proteomic core facility. In fact, the money for the position comes from the proteomic facility and so running that unit is job #1.

So far, one candidate is favored by most of the faculty. She has a history of R01 funding, and in her seminar she was innovative and seen as intellectually ahead of the other candidates.

In your discussions with her, she says she is happy where she is and has put up some big numbers to make it worthwhile for her to move. Her request for lab space exceeds the allotment of others of her rank, and her request for a discretionary fund of $1M (to allegedly make up what monies she would need to leave behind) also exceeds what others of like position have. Otherwise, the number of new positions she would like is available within the package you have, and her equipment requirements are already within the proteomic facility. However, you are getting a bit concerned that she has raised no issues with regard to what would be expected of her in the role of director of the proteomic facility.

You have spoken with colleagues at her home institution. She is uniformly described as bright with a high IQ. Some say she is very direct and gets right in your face in personal debates. One commented that she doesn't suffer fools.

You are thinking she would be fine as a faculty member, but you are not sure how she would be as director of the proteomic facility. The problem is that the package for the proteomic facility came from a donor, and he wants a star in that position.

Negotiating begins with an understanding of the other parties and their interests (and your own interests).

What would you do?

© Springer International Publishing Switzerland 2015
J.L. Houpt et al., *Learning to Lead in the Academic Medical Center*,
DOI 10.1007/978-3-319-21260-9_19

Chapter 20
Dr. Un Settled: Negotiation and Middle-Age Dysphoria

Dr. Un Settled is a tenured associate professor in infectious diseases, and her name has just begun to be circulated as a potential division head candidate at a few well-respected programs. She has been happy in her current position but would like something more. While being successful in maintaining grant support, she feels overwhelmed by the prospect of having to keep doing this for another 20 or more years. She feels the pace is just too much. Also she was recently put on some medical school-wide committees and found herself pleasantly surprised at enjoying thinking at that level. She has always been a mentor and has enjoyed that part of her job. Her current division head has no intention of giving up the job.

Un Settled has a spouse who is a pediatrician in a large practice in town. Fortunately he has a malpractice tail and could move. She has two children, one who is a senior in high school and going off to college next year and another who is a rising junior in high school.

A friend and colleague of hers in gastroenterology, of similar age and academic progression, was recently offered a division head position at an outstanding institution. He turned it down when his current division head made a retention offer which involved a raise, a travel allowance, a promise to help him achieve center designation, and an initiation of steps for consideration of an early promotion. She'd be happy to find a similar solution.

This is not the first retention offer made recently. In fact, the chair of the department was recently retained with a significant financial package to rebuild the department, when he was a finalist for a dean's position. She hates the idea of interviewing in order to get an offer but believes, as do many others, that currently at least you have to get an outside offer to get what you would like to achieve here.

Un Settled seeks your advice.

How would you advise Dr. Un Settled?

© Springer International Publishing Switzerland 2015
J.L. Houpt et al., *Learning to Lead in the Academic Medical Center*,
DOI 10.1007/978-3-319-21260-9_20

Chapter 21
Dr. Green, Conflict Resolution, and Managing Up and Down

Dr. Green has served six months as chair of surgery. The dean had appointed him as an outside candidate over the strenuous objections of the powerful previous chair, Dr. Black, a vascular surgeon. Dr. Black had lobbied hard, though unsuccessfully, for his protégé in the division of vascular surgery and division chief, Dr. Cole, to succeed him as chair. Dr. Black has been actively undermining Dr. Green's efforts to bring greater harmony to a highly fractured department and to substantially increase revenues and improve a generally anemic research base in the department, all of which he had been charged to do by the dean when he was appointed.

Revenues from vascular surgery in particular are at risk because of intense competition in the surrounding markets. As a solution, the division of vascular surgery, led by Drs. Cole and his mentor, Dr. Black, has been fighting hard to separate themselves from general surgery and to form a separate department of vascular and endovascular surgery. They apparently made a reasonable and legitimate, though not compelling, clinical and business case for doing so. Other divisions are strongly opposed.

The announcement by another prominent medical school in the state that they have created a new department of vascular and endovascular surgery has inflamed the vascular surgery faculty, who are now irate that their already-declining competitive position will be compromised further by the other school's announcement and enhanced visibility. They demand a joint meeting with Dr. Green and the dean.

What would you do?

© Springer International Publishing Switzerland 2015
J.L. Houpt et al., *Learning to Lead in the Academic Medical Center*,
DOI 10.1007/978-3-319-21260-9_21

Chapter 22
Drs. Rich and Pure: Conflict of Interest (COI) and Creating School-Wide Policies

In the past decade, the power within the department of medicine has resided in the division of cardiology. The division is heavily involved in industry-funded clinical trials as well as clinical care. The division's faculty has extensive ties with industry, including lucrative speaking engagements, training programs for other cardiologists, particularly in the procedural subspecialties, and three start-up companies built around various cardiac devices invented by division faculty along with surgery faculty. NIH funding for the department has declined in the past three years but is still relatively strong in relation to other departments of medicine nationally.

Last year, there was a scandal within the cardiology division that reverberated through the school and university. It involved a nationally prominent professor in the cardiology division, Dr. Rich, with large, active NIH grants, who failed to report on his annual conflicts of interest disclosure $500,000 in consulting fees from speaking engagements at a major pharma company. His NIH grants involve two compounds in which the company is interested. The fallout from NIH was serious.

Dr. Pure, also a professor in the division, has written extensively on the topic of physician/industry relationships, arguing that there should be no personal financial interests with industry and no CME funding from industry. He has a strong following among the fellows and students but not among other faculty. The local papers as well as the national press have editorialized on the subject of pharma and device companies buying prominent figures in academic medicine. The university's Board of Trustees has demanded that conflicts of interest be cleaned up. At the same time, they have urged the university administration to aggressively pursue industry funding of research as well as industry gifts for the university's new capital campaign.

There is a new dean of the school who has been in place for six months. She has brought you in as the new chair of medicine from a private institution, where you were chief of cardiology. She wants you to lead the effort to clean up the

© Springer International Publishing Switzerland 2015   157
J.L. Houpt et al., *Learning to Lead in the Academic Medical Center*,
DOI 10.1007/978-3-319-21260-9_22

relationships with industry, but she is conscious of the need to retain strong, nationally prominent faculty and good relationships with industry (the source of increasing industry support for clinical trials). Ideally, she wants you to "cinch down," school wide, on personal relationships with industry while keeping everybody happy. She would like for you to enlist the support of other chairs so that the effort can be made to "stick" school wide.

What would you do?

Chapter 23
Budget Cuts and Managing Bad News and Incentivizing Faculty

You are the new chair of a clinical department in the medical school. One of your initial efforts is to create a departmental compensation plan. You create a task force, which works for nearly a year on a new plan, balancing out appropriate rewards for clinical, research, and other mission-related productivity. The plan includes a baseline salary, which is to be the median salary for that specialty, role (clinical versus research), and rank based on national data from the prior three years. An incentive plan includes payments for RVUs generated in excess of the median benchmark, along with incentives for funding of research effort and other mission/citizenship work. In the end, there is enthusiasm for the plan because many faculty will see increases in salary, as faculty below national means will see annual raises of the maximum allowable percent until their salaries reach the appropriate level. For some faculty, this would require 3–5 years of annual raises, given that current salaries are so low.

Less than one year later, the state cuts funding to the School of Medicine (SOM). The dean sends an email to all the departments and faculty. In it he says that the SOM must reduce its expenditures by $8M to accommodate the decrease in state funding. He points out that there will be personnel and non-personnel expense reductions in the dean's office and encourages departments to do the same. He sends out specific expense reduction targets by department.

Since this memo was sent from the dean's office to the entire faculty, you quickly learn that the following attitudes and concerns are right on the surface with the faculty:

1. Several members of the department have undergone nonrenewals of their contracts in the last 5 years, including faculty who were perceived by their peers to have done good work. This caused significant problems with overall departmental morale at the time, and those effects are still lingering. Additionally, fixed-term faculty are beginning to wonder if they too are at risk.
2. Other faculty members are counting on the raises that were promised to them as part of the faculty compensation plan. Although the fine print of the plan states

© Springer International Publishing Switzerland 2015
J.L. Houpt et al., *Learning to Lead in the Academic Medical Center*,
DOI 10.1007/978-3-319-21260-9_23

that its implementation is contingent on state funding, the faculty heard you promise raises.

3. Your faculty note that the memo from the dean addresses only reduction of expenses, not increasing revenue. They argue that reducing the numbers of faculty members will reduce income, which is a goal seemingly contradictory to the vision of the department (and the reason you were hired) to stimulate growth. Reducing support staff will decrease efficiency and therefore also reduce productivity, income, and growth. They want you to go to the dean and argue against expense reduction in favor of revenue generation.

You also meet with the dean's budget people and with your own and find out that your department's share of the cuts is 3 % of your personnel budget, which, together with the 6 % increase in budget that was necessary to get all the pay raises accomplished, gives you a new 9 % hole.

How would you think through this dilemma and determine your cuts and how would you communicate it to the faculty?

What would you do?

Chapter 24
A "No-Brainer": Dr. Virtue Comes to State University Medical Center

Dr. Virtue (Dr. V) has recently been appointed to be the new chair of the department of medicine at State University Medical Center (SUMC). He was brought in from outside, having served as the vice chair of his previous department. Shortly after arriving, he was approached by Associate Dean Dr. Do Good with a request to help sponsor an initiative called "The Code of Conduct." The "Code" is a set of rules or principles designed to promote positive collegial relationships across the medical center. This initiative came about because of several reported incidents of bullying and harassment in the institution. The other driver of this initiative was the most recent physician satisfaction scores from SUMC. The survey measures physician engagement and their perceived quality of work life and collegiality. SUMC placed in the bottom quartile of this national survey.

The Code of Conduct was designed to serve as a set of operating principles to address the problem of what was increasingly described as a hostile work environment and to ensure that people treat one another with respect, refrain from any abusive or intimidating behavior, and promote a positive culture of cooperation. Dr. V was very positive about this initiative. In addition, his prior institution had enacted a similar program called "Rules of the Road," which provided a set of detailed guidelines as a code of conduct.

Dr. V began to champion the program immediately. At one of his first faculty meetings, Dr. V asked the Associate Dean Do Good to present this initiative and field questions the faculty might have. Dr. V was somewhat surprised at the lack of positive reception on the part of his colleagues and the lack of any discussion after Dr. Do Good's presentation. Nevertheless, he proceeded with his plan and appointed a committee (the Culture Taskforce) of respected senior faculty to take the Code, customize it for the department of medicine, and plan how to implement its use as a tool for faculty, staff, and student performance evaluations. While he had some difficulty getting some of the physicians to agree to serve on the task force, he attributed their reluctance to the usual challenge of getting busy physicians to engage in service activities. Dr. V was convinced that this initiative would support his broader objective of making the department of medicine a center of excellence, distinguished

© Springer International Publishing Switzerland 2015
J.L. Houpt et al., *Learning to Lead in the Academic Medical Center*,
DOI 10.1007/978-3-319-21260-9_24

by its positive culture and productive work environment for research, teaching, and clinical service.

Six months later, when Dr. V is in his sixth month of tenure as chair, he sees clear signs of progress in some areas, but he is disturbed by a lack of progress in his efforts to develop a more positive departmental culture. He was realistic, he thought, about the likelihood of some resistance, but he did not expect the overt challenge and hostility communicated by his colleagues (particularly ones who he had seen as his support base). He knew there was a lot of behind-the-scenes talk among senior faculty about being on a "forced march," which was part of a larger backlash against what many faculty saw as the imposition of a business-driven corporate culture.

As Dr. V was to learn, the backlash was a response to SUMC's top management's efforts to bring business practices and discipline to the AMC. The CEO of SUMC Healthcare and her high-level administrators brought a different bottom-line-oriented perspective to the institution. They communicated a clear message about efficiency, cutting costs, and generating revenue. This message was followed by the administration's strong efforts to enforce compliance with new metrics and processes designed to make financial management and discipline the order of the day.

After several members of the Culture Taskforce had resigned in protest over what they saw as yet another example of being "corporatized" *and* infantilized ("telling us how to behave"), Dr. V had to appoint some junior (but tenured) faculty. They were more supportive of the effort, and on a number of key issues they moved things forward for a while by outvoting their senior colleagues. This led to thinly veiled threats by their senior colleagues and protests about the "tyranny of the majority." As the rancor increased, the younger faculty members' support for the Code began to waver. At this point, Dr. V muses, the net effect of the culture change effort is negative—it has spawned a divisive, adversarial backlash that threatens to undermine every cooperative initiative he wants to initiate in the department.

Dr. V has no idea what to do to get his efforts on track. He wonders why a program of such obvious importance and value flounders so badly. What should he have done to prevent this adverse outcome? How could he have anticipated this reaction? What can he do to turn things around?

What would you do?

Part V
Teaching Materials

Each of the chapters in this part begins with a repetition of one of the cases in Part IV, including the open-ended question that concludes each of those cases, but then we add to each case certain materials that we think may be helpful for the teacher or discussion leader. The materials consist, first, of our view in a nutshell of what each case is about. These summaries are provided as a means for the teacher to take advantage if he/she chooses of our experience in actually using these cases with a succession of classes of leaders and emerging leaders. Following the nutshell summary of each case, we then offer specific questions that we have used to prompt group discussion on what we consider to be the important issues in each case. We note the particular substantive points that we intend to elicit as a means to help the teacher keep the discussion on track and focused on the key issues each case is designed to illustrate.

Chapter 25
Strategic Planning/Outside Consultants: Power and Authority, Vertical Hierarchies, and the Informal Organization

The university chancellor, with blessings from the Board of Trustees, initiated a comprehensive, 2-year, university-wide strategic planning process that included the medical school. A large and prestigious national consulting firm was hired to help, and there followed a broad, open, 18-month process, out of which emerged a strategic plan with components for each school or college, including the medical school. Several members of the medical school faculty and the then dean of medicine served on key committees established as parts of the planning process that led up to the strategic plan itself.

Halfway through the planning process, the then dean developed serious health problems and resigned from his post, thus causing the chancellor to undertake a search for a new dean. Following a national search with participation from across the medical school, Dr. Rose, a well-known clinician/researcher and chair of the department of medicine at a prestigious New England Medical School, was hired with great anticipation. During his meetings with the search committee, the strategic plan was actively and supportively discussed. In Dr. Rose's negotiations with the chancellor, a key part of the chancellor's expectations and charge to him was to implement the medical school's portion of the strategic plan, which the chancellor and the trustees enthusiastically embraced, as did the new dean. A principal component of the plan involved the strategic acquisition of two well-located hospitals in the medical school's market area, as well as a number of clinical practices, so as to produce both a more integrated and more distributed system, better able to absorb the challenges associated with the redesign of the American healthcare system.

Since the plan was the product of broad input from faculty and staff across the university, was widely publicized, and was endorsed by the former dean, Dr. Rose immediately established an implementation committee to initiate the steps necessary to move forward with the plan's recommendations on hospital and practice acquisitions.

Immediately after the first steps were taken, all hell breaks loose in the press, which characterizes the initiatives as "anticompetitive," "predatory," and "grasping." The faculty expresses great consternation in the halls and clinics of the school

© Springer International Publishing Switzerland 2015
J.L. Houpt et al., *Learning to Lead in the Academic Medical Center*,
DOI 10.1007/978-3-319-21260-9_25

and in faculty meetings, and it quickly becomes apparent to Dr. Rose that there is no internal or external consensus on the plan. Meanwhile, the chancellor and the trustees are expecting quarterly progress reports on implementation of the plan from the various deans, including the new medical school dean.

What would you do?

The case in a nutshell is this: in this case, the group usually sees Dr. Rose as victim and the consultants and university leadership as the culprits, who achieved what the chancellor and trustees wanted all along. The case presents a scenario that challenges the new dean's understanding of the power and limits of vertical hierarchies and crucial role of the informal organization (Chap. 1). It also demonstrates the difference between authority and power (Chap. 3). When a leader is given a mandate as here, it is based on the power and decision-making rights of the formal organization. What is critical to keep in mind is that formal rights are only a necessary but not sufficient basis for making decisions that can be implemented. You as dean, chair, or division head have formal decision-making rights, but such rights are meaningless if you do not get support and buy-in from the informal organization. The latter is an invisible but powerful force in all organizations, especially in academic institutions where the most entrenched interests are tenured or politically protected. There are no leaders without followers. And those followers, individuals, and groups reside in the informal organization, which must be reckoned with, influenced, and motivated to support the leader's vision and direction.

This case is complicated by Dr. Rose's instruction to act quickly—before he has a chance to earn his authority from the faculty (Chap. 3). Further, he's in the middle between the faculty and the chancellor and trustees, and the facts as presented draw into question whether he can convince the faculty that as their leader he can ensure their survival. He should have anticipated the faculty response and dealt with it in the process of being hired. He didn't. The solution requires quickly aligning the village elders and others with the vision of those who have bought into the plan.

What assumptions about power and authority, vertical hierarchies, and formal and informal organizations were made by Dr. Rose and the chancellor?

This was a top-down process driven by the Board of Trustees and the chancellor, using the outside consulting firm to create a strategic plan. It assumes that vertical hierarchies (Chap. 1) can effectively create change. It ignores the expertise of those in the lower ranks who know the day-to-day realities in the clinical market place. The case also illustrates organizational leadership that fails to understand and utilize the informal organization, particularly the village elders (Chap. 1). The university leadership relies on the dean's power to effect change, but it ignores the fact that he had not yet earned the authority to effect so bold a move (Chap. 3). In short, university leadership appears to have made the incorrect assumption that the AMC is just like any other business where a board can set direction and executives can execute the plan (Chap. 2). Dr. Rose assumed that because there were faculty on the strategic planning committee, it was blessed by all the faculty.

What does the planning process say about the culture of the medical school? The university? Is it different from a business? If you think it is, how would you explain it to a business person on the board?

This case provides an opportunity to consider if and how a university is different from a business. There is no single or correct answer. Some believe that medical schools are businesses that have been run poorly. Further, some believe that for a medical school to be run properly, proven business principles should be followed.

Others think medical schools are more like a sports teams or opera companies than normal businesses. While these are businesses, the emphasis is on the players or performers. They have prima donnas and divas, and the players are not interchangeable, so the enterprises have to constantly adapt to the ego needs of the players. The businesses don't run the divas; the businesses are organized around the divas and their needs (Robert Michels and Jeff Houpt, personal communication).

Some also take the entrepreneurial/biotech approach and argue that the AMC is like a biotech company where many ideas are funded in order to find a truly innovative one. Thus, loss is a precondition of gain. Such a business can't stand too much loss before it sees gain.

Whatever view is taken by those who are not a part of the AMC, the planning process in this case ran into trouble because it was top down. In a medical school, how you do what you do is as important as what you do. This is particularly true in "process" schools but also true to some degree in "executive" schools (Chap. 2). This value of process is one key way a medical school differs from most businesses.

By the time an individual is a candidate to be a dean, he or she should have a sense about how to use consultants and their potential benefits and costs, especially large consulting firms. How are they viewed by faculty, and when and how should an individual leader use consultants?

Boards of Trustees are often made up of successful businessmen/businesswomen who have had to move their organization into new waters. To do so, they use name brand consultants, create plans with significant communication components to build buy-in, and then in essence begin a companywide conversion process. They understand that it is a massive effort, and they often use big-name firms to help to get it done.

The faculty meanwhile are skeptical at best, but more likely cynical. When big firms ask for faculty "input," they often know that their input has little effect. Their view may be that the outcome has already been determined by the board, the chancellor, and the highly paid consultants who are expert at giving back to the board the recommendations that they want.

> An example from my experience illustrates the point. I was called by a member of the search committee to vet a candidate they were looking at a possible dean. She wanted to know if the candidate was naïve or not. I asked why that had come up, and she replied that they had just had a well-known firm in to develop a strategic plan and they had just made their recommendations on priorities. "What I want to know is whether the candidate knows to mouth these priorities to the President while at the same time understanding they don't fit the school. They don't represent our strengths or protect our niche – they're just the most lucrative from a business standpoint," she asked.

Thus, one way to view this case is that Dr. Rose, instead of being cast as a victim, should have known the skepticism that faculty might have toward the consultants and university leadership. Since he didn't, it would draw into question whether he could meet the first responsibility of the group leader—to protect the group. We will talk below about how he might have handled it.

However, despite faculty cynicism, consulting firms have an important place, particularly in two instances. First, if you have to make a change that is major and will be controversial and thus is a change that may exceed your capacity to persuade, either time-wise or emotionally, you may want to use an outside consulting firm. And, second, if you become convinced that you must do something and you don't believe that you can get the troops to buy into it, you might want to use a big firm. That is exactly what happened above. The trustees weren't convinced that the deans could get the job done and so they got a consultant to recommend the changes they wanted. The Board of Trustees approved the recommendations from the consultant. They got to where they wanted to be by using power, not authority. If you use this approach, you just need to understand that you have not gotten buy-in. You will have to work on that aspect after the fact.

For most of your everyday work, however, power tactics and big-name firms are not needed. It is far more prudent to use the informal organization and other strategies to build buy-in.

With the benefit of hindsight, what might Dr. Rose have done?

If Dr. Rose were not so naïve, he would have suspected that there was resistance to the plan, even though he was being told it was accepted and finalized. If the trustees were cognizant of the culture in the AMC, they would have chosen a candidate who was skeptical and a bit cynical. But more than likely, they chose someone who assured them that he bought into the plan and was the one to implement it. In fact, it was probably a precondition of being picked. Remember, the chancellor and board are expecting quarterly reports. Any candidate questioning the support for the plan could potentially look indecisive and wimpy. One approach that Dr. Rose might have taken would be to question faculty in private about the plan. He could have asked to return to campus for an extra visit and talk to those within the school about the plan, rather than just to rely on the representation to the planning process that had been put into place before his arrival. If he had done that, he would likely have found out that there was no buy-in.

Let's assume that Dr. Rose did make that extra visit and learned of the faculty's resistance. He then needs to decide if he backs the plan or not-or alternatively, what he backs and what he is not sure of. He then needs to meet with the chancellor and board chair. Demeanor is crucial here. He needs to be confident and aggressive because the chancellor and board chair could read his concerns as a weakness and dismiss his comments. He needs to speak with authority and assurance. They have to be convinced that he is on top of things and that even though the message is not what they want to hear, he is the one to trust.

Here's what he might say. "I know you had a university-wide process to develop this plan, and it had two (for example) members of the medical school on it and the former dean. The dean is no longer here so you have a plan bought into by two people. That's it, you have the endorsement of two – yet there are 1400 faculty over there." (You pause; see Chap. 11 on Mastering the Art of Persuasion.)

They say for him to proceed anyway. He responds "Ok, so I exaggerated a little, but not much because we have no idea how many will support this and how many will not. The good news is that I support it, (if you don't, then you shouldn't have taken the job), and as you know I came back and spent two extra days talking to the busiest clinicians and researchers, and I think they will support it with some caveats. But several think it's a violation of our mission and a sellout to corporate greed and are prepared to go to the local paper."

"So here's the deal from my point of view – I like it and I'm prepared to work towards its implementation. But there will be resistance – it might get public – and I need to know if you are going to support me at that time. One final thing, if you give me six months to sell it, I can diminish the backlash, and even though I can't eliminate it, I can lessen it. That's it – what do you think?"

Chapter 26
Dr. Newby: Change, Getting Started, and Your Baby Is Ugly

You have just been named the chair of a clinical department at the medical school of the people. You came from a prestigious private medical school. Your charge by the dean is to increase the research presence of the department and school.

Brimming with confidence, you are offered a reasonable package but the state is going through a recession, state funding is decreasing, and third-party reimbursements are decreasing. Nevertheless, you start recruiting aggressively. Meanwhile, members of the department are talking in whispers about the wisdom of your pursuing these external recruitments when their compensation is threatened. A small chorus of faculty start saying out loud that maybe you ought to be using your package to bolster their income and not using it on outside people at least until things turn around economically.

Move forward a few weeks: two faculty come to see you to tell you that they are making plans to leave the department and to set up a practice in town, which of course will be in direct competition with the department. Also, these two people are the franchise, and if they leave, you will need to recruit new people to replace them.

You receive considerable counsel from the departmental faculty to retain these people but you have troubles from a number of points. They do not do research, and their field is one in which there are a pool of clinician/scientists.

So the area is high on your list as one in which you can meet the dean's charge to increase the research dollars. Even more disconcerting to you is that you do not consider the people you're asked to retain to be hard workers and in fact have concluded recently that you must put in a more incentive-laden compensation plan in order to get faculty working harder.

You permit the individuals to leave without any counter offer and form a committee to review the compensation plan. You charge the committee to look specifically at the department's incentives, and you provide them with a consulting firm to assist in getting national data as norms for work effort.

Move forward one year: three more faculty have left and your first two recruits have just joined your faculty. They are first rate and to get them you had to offer them more in salary than the existing faculty and give them the best space. You are

© Springer International Publishing Switzerland 2015   171
J.L. Houpt et al., *Learning to Lead in the Academic Medical Center*,
DOI 10.1007/978-3-319-21260-9_26

really pleased with them and have started three more searches. You are unaware of how these recruits are viewed. While you view them as great additions that everyone will welcome, they are instead seen by the existing faculty as evidence that you don't respect the existing people and the careers they have had.

Meanwhile, your committee on compensation is ready to report out and you receive a lackluster report that has something for every constituent but no real driving incentives and no robust benchmarks that you had hoped for. You talk to the committee chair, whom you handpicked, and he tells you that the committee was divided between those with a view like yours ("eat what you kill") and those concerned with tradition ("the plan needs to pay for teaching and citizenship and not just research and clinical work" which you interpret to mean "if we wanted to work that hard we'd have gone into private practice").

You get a call from the dean/CEO to tell you that he got a call from an important legislator who wanted to know "what is going on there." It appears that one of your department's faculty is the physician for this legislator, and he hears that you are driving away all the teachers in favor of researchers and bringing in all your own people from outside. The dean suggests that you need to show some interest in the old-timers. He makes it pretty clear that he wants everybody happy.

You leave the dean's office and wonder how you are going to handle this. Surely, if you side with the "eat what you kill group," it will get back to the legislator. If you confront the physician to the legislator, you could be charged with retaliation. If you don't put in the new compensation plan, you will never get the salaries up and your precious resources will be spent on the status quo. You have two really good recruits and potentially three on the line. If you get them, you are well on your way to having a transformed and terrific department. From your perspective, you are being asked to back off and support mediocrity, yet that is not what the dean told you when he hired you.

What would you do?

The case in a nutshell is this: we begin by letting the group freelance on how they would approach this case. Most see the critical nature of Dr. Newby, and many relate to the compensation committee report because they have been involved recently in developing new compensation plans.

This case presents one of the most common situations that new chairs find themselves in-the need to move into a new area or upgrade an old one. Can the chair do it while keeping the faculty positively involved or will she drive them away and into an oppositional mode? The chair needs to find a way to honor the people and achievements of the past while promoting change by (1) helping existing faculty members adapt and expand their roles and contributions as much as possible and (2) bringing in new faculty to strengthen the research portfolio of the department. The leader's role here is to balance the need for the organization to preserve the key elements of the past (the purpose and values of an academic department) while promoting new capabilities and innovation as energetically as possible. While this might seem like mission impossible, it is in fact the key challenge all leaders must play if they are to build and sustain successful organizations. Once a leader understands this, he/she needs to find a way to frame and communicate the both/and agenda so that everyone who should be a part of the new future understands their role and the legitimacy and importance of everyone else's. Once you know who you want to stay on board, there can be no winners or losers; otherwise, internal strife will irreparably damage the department and deplete its resources.

If the group has mentioned Dr. Newby's critical nature, a natural segue into the case is as follows.

Putting aside the personality issues, what are the different parties' interests in this case?

One way to view this scenario is to view it as a clash of personalities— Dr. Newby's extremely critical nature and the department's recalcitrance (passive–aggressive response, to some). But, as we suggested in Chap. 13, you'd be wise to put that aside and just view the contrasting interests. Dr. Newby has a certain definition of excellence and work ethic that she would like to instill. The department has a sense of cohesion, work expectations, and definition of excellence from the past that they want to keep.

Two factors have complicated the situation. First, Dr. Newby has convinced the group that she does not respect them. Recall she tries to fire a resident, lets two faculty go without an attempt to retain them, and has hired a consultant to redesign the compensation plan because they are "lazy." Second, the dean and legislator are now watching, so Dr. Newby is now on the defensive.

One of the hardest arguments to make in the AMC is to tell people that they are not perfect and that there is room for improvement, largely because their self-esteem depends on opposite feelings about their intellects. Consequently, entreaties meant to say "We need to get better" are seen as declarations that "Your baby is ugly." How do you avoid this?

There is hardly any circumstance when you need to say that "your baby is ugly." A wise person would anticipate those circumstances, that is, when your message might be heard that way, and take steps to avoid their drawing of that conclusion. You simply must express appreciation for the work that they do while affirming the need to move forward in some areas.

The most successful leaders (and most successful people in general) find something to like in everyone. They relate to that likeable characteristic and thus can carry on an honest admiration for the person while continuing to hold a critical opinion of other characteristics. Said alternatively, they don't see people as all good or all bad.

People know if you despise them. If you ever drive home at night convinced that you are surrounded by fools, you've lost your ability to lead. Take a break. Come back when you still are frustrated to death by them but haven't given up on them.

What plan would you develop for each of these players: faculty, compensation committee, dean, and legislator?

One approach would be to meet with each of these people individually before calling for a faculty meeting. You could start anywhere but we'd start with the dean.

Keep it simple with the dean. Get your argument down to a sentence, paragraph, and page, as described in Chap. 11. There are two issues to deal with: (1) the assertion by the legislator that you are opposed to teaching and (2) the unhappiness of the faculty with the decisions that you have made.

With regard to the assertion that you are opposed to teaching, you must make a declarative statement that nothing is further from the truth. You must always forcefully oppose any statements putting you on the wrong side of core values. If the teaching ratings of your recent recruits are good, show them to him. If you don't have them, you make the argument that these recruits will raise the reputation of the department and lead to better residents and a better teaching program. But most importantly, argue with passion about how you will support education. You can then ask the dean if he would like you to talk to the legislator.

The issue of collateral damage and the dean's injunction to make everybody happy needs to be dealt with. Obviously, making everybody happy is impossible, but we wouldn't raise that. Deans don't like to look silly. One approach is this: "I'm sorry about the discontent. I can see now that I might have handled things differently. But I don't regret recruiting these new people and letting the others go. This department is significantly better than it was when I came and is close to meeting the standard that we talked about when I took the job. I can see that I didn't explain where I was going enough and didn't get enough feedback and buy-in. I'm going to try to correct that."

Such an approach may do it for the dean. It gives him a way to save face with the legislator. "I talked with Dr. Newby and she convinced me that she does favor education. But she made some changes without enough consensus. She readily admits her mistakes and assures me that she will work on correcting them."

Obviously, you could have taken the approach with the dean that you both agreed on this and he has to support you. That's the righteous, indignant, and principled approach. We'd recommend against it. When you are in a pickle with your boss, and you are not entirely blameless, it's far shrewder to admit improprieties in process and set about to correct them. When arguing for his support when you have made mistakes, it is far better to admit your errors than asking him to overlook them as a matter of principle.

Compensation committee. One way to start is to tell them you want to understand the reasoning behind their recommendations. Once again, this is a negotiation, and so the first job is to understand the interests behind their recommendations (i.e., their positions) (see Chap. 8).

We'd begin this way. "What I want to do today is to report on my meeting with the dean, and then I want to spend the rest of the time hearing your thoughts about the compensation plan." Then you proceed to tell them that the meeting with the dean went well, how passionate you are about education, and that you readily acknowledge that you had not done enough consulting with them and getting their input—and that you told the dean that as well. (Two things are accomplished by beginning with the dean. One, you've told them that you have him back on your side. And second, you've given them an apology and challenged them to step up to the plate and help you.)

At this point, it's important to step back and let them talk. Don't respond to every statement. Continue to ask for more. We'd let it go 30 min before interrupting. It can go one of two ways. The worst is 30 min of hostile complaining with no real suggestions out of the situation. In that case, it is useful to just say, calmly, "Okay, I've heard you. Now, concretely, what would you want me to do?" This is the best way we can think of to get back on a problem-solving track (see Chap. 12). If the group is not so hostile, you listen to them and restate your case, making sure that you deal with their interests. More than likely, they will say, "We want things the way they were." You, on the other hand, will want to go to "While it worked in the past, we need to change." You then need to make the case for why the survival of the group requires that they change. The most common way to do this to point out that the only way to ensure them competitive compensation in the future is to tighten up the compensation plan—that it is for the good and survival of the group.

Faculty. By this time the dean and the compensation committee may have come around. In meeting with the faculty, you need to go over the ground you covered with the dean, especially owning up to mistakes in process and passionately supporting education. You assert your interest in consulting with them in the future. Then you present a vision of a department as being on the threshold of being included among the best.

What role does the feeling that Dr. Newby doesn't respect the current faculty play in this?

In our experience, it has everything to do with coups. It is what gives the energy to revolts. It is a form of group narcissistic injury. (see Chap. 4 on Narcissism).

With the benefit of hindsight, do this over again.

Begin with buy-in from the faculty, not just the dean (faculty meetings, one on ones, listen sessions, committees)—all the issues in Chap. 3 on Authority Is Earned, Not Bestowed and Chap. 7 on Getting Started the Right Way.

Involve the dean in discussions of collateral damage as soon as they happen. Never let him be surprised and find out from a legislator. Remember all the players in a change scenario—bosses, village elders, mafia, and then faculty. Meet with them, listen, and get them on board; then move.

One final caveat. Dr. Newby could rescue herself if she had the interpersonal skills to so it. She would need to truly respect some of what they do, and not be so critical. They would need to feel that she liked them and didn't disdain them. The case illustrates the importance of personality factors in determining success or failure.

Chapter 27
Dr. Worksalot: Personality and Getting Started

Dr. Worksalot (Dr. W) was named chair of a clinical department one and one-half years ago. The dean selected him because his academic credentials were superior to anyone in the department, and the dean had fond hopes that Dr. W could add a much-needed NIH presence to the mostly clinical department. Early on, Dr. W. noted that the residents were not of a caliber acceptable to him, and, likewise, a couple of the faculty in his opinion should be released. He tried to energize the residency director to oust a resident at the year's end, but the residency director produced repeated evaluations showing that the resident did "acceptable" to more than "expected" work. The residency committee rejected the new chair's request.

Dr. W happened to be an introvert and perfectionist, as well as a workaholic. This had been no problem in his meteoric rise as an academic because he could retreat to his lab and just work harder whenever stressed or when in jeopardy of losing his grant. This didn't bother his students and postdocs because they didn't expect much socializing or even basic social niceties. His reputation as borderline Asperger's didn't bother them either. They signed up despite that because they respected his IQ. Even though he was a taskmaster, it was no problem—his postdocs got jobs. It didn't matter that he never complimented them and needed endless data to make a decision. They didn't care because they preferred getting great training and a job to a warm and cuddly boss.

But the faculty didn't respond like his students. When the dean heard grumblings of dissatisfaction with Dr. W from the faculty, he hired a coach for him. The coach suggested that he "get out and around" and get to know people and show an interest in them instead of staying holed up in his office and sending out peremptory memos. Dr. W did as suggested. He reported the meetings a "great success." However, the faculty and residents who Dr. W visited felt as if they were "graded" on their responses to his inquiries and then found him lacking.

At the end of year one, he let an assistant professor go because he didn't believe the junior person was up to his standards. The person he let go was a protégée of a much respected member of the department who had actually served one year as chief of the medical staff. Dr W doubted the value of the mentor as well.

© Springer International Publishing Switzerland 2015
J.L. Houpt et al., *Learning to Lead in the Academic Medical Center*,
DOI 10.1007/978-3-319-21260-9_27

By a year and a half, members of the faculty were grumbling about their new chair.

What would you advise Dr. Worksalot to do?

The case in a nutshell is this: in our experience, most classes have focused on Dr. W's personality, especially his huge introversion and his perfectionism. That is entirely appropriate, as this case is about personality traits that derail performance. In our classes, we often pair this case with a discussion of the Myers–Briggs (Chap. 4), and have the class take the test online and then bring their printout to class to discuss.

With respect to Dr. W's extreme introversion, does he have the interpersonal capacity to rescue himself, or is he too damaged to change? And does he need to look for a vice chair to supply the necessary interpersonal skills (Chap. 4)? We suggest that one way to make that determination is to describe the actions he would need to take to turn this around and assess whether he is capable of taking them.

The case also opens up two additional questions. First, what are the skills required to get promoted and what are those required to deal successfully with the responsibilities of higher positions? It highlights that a candidate's success depends on the ability to make the transition from individual contributor to a builder of organizations and the psychological capacity to develop an altruistic approach to his or her career (Chap. 6).

Finally, the case provides an opportunity to explore whether you need to recruit a researcher to build a research program and whether you need a clinician to build a clinical program.

What is the role of personality in leadership? Define Dr. W's shortcomings. Do you see any strengths? Is there any way to compensate for his shortcomings?

We made the case in Chap. 4 that having personality shortcomings is not lethal in its own right if you can find a way to compensate for them. However, Dr. W's shortcomings look potentially derailing. The fact that he was described as borderline Asperger's suggests that his introversion is severe (review Chap. 4 on introversion and its problems here). There is also the problem of his narcissism as it's expressed in his criticism of others and in his sense that no one in the room measures up to him.

There are, however, some strengths. From his time with postdocs and students, we see an individual that is bright, can mentor (in the right context), and can go out of his way to help people get jobs. Thus, he can be generative. The problem is that it seems to require a subservient master/student relationship to carry it off (review Chap. 15 on why we pick the wrong people and the section on eliminating personality disorders, Appendix A, and Appendix B).

In Chap. 4 on Personality Traits and Leadership, we speak of compensating for shortcomings. One approach here might be to look at using other people to compensate for Dr. W's extreme introversion instead of trying to get him to change. Dr. W could find a highly respected member of the department who was there before he came and make that person a vice chair. This new vice chair would do the talking, the brokering, and the explaining and would involve the faculty as peers in the process. Dr. W would become chief strategist and build the external reputation by being active at national meetings and in national organizations. This could be a stretch in terms of whether that would be enough, but Dr. W would have a better chance of succeeding than he would on his own.

Can Dr. W salvage his situation and, as his adviser, what would you recommend?

We would assess Dr. W's situation as difficult to salvage. He may not be fired, but, unless he changes his ways, he probably would not be renewed at year 5. Fundamentally, Dr. W has to find a way to start over. He needs to acknowledge his mistakes and apologize. And, in our opinion, he needs to accept the idea of a vice chair to compensate for his shortcomings. Others may feel differently and see an opportunity to change, but our verdict would be the opposite. Either way, we need to ask what he should do. And if we think we know the answer to that question, we then need to ask whether he could do it.

Our approach would be this. We'd recommend that he stand before the departmental faculty and say it's obvious that "I started off on the wrong foot. I'd like to start over today by outlining my vision for the department and seek your feedback both on it and on ways that I can do better. First of all, I want a department that honors not just research but clinical work and teaching as well. I see our field at a most exciting time. This is the time for our field, and I desperately want us to participate in it. I have great respect for the traditions of the department and the contributions of all who went before me. I took the job because I wanted to build on that. Unfortunately, in my haste to move us forward, I did so in a way that implied that I didn't respect what was here. That was due to my haste and my passion – but that is not an adequate excuse, and so I apologize."

If he agrees with our idea of a vice chair, he continues, "I have asked (long time member of the department) to assist me by becoming an executive vice chair. H/she will be leading an effort to chart our forward motion, and I promise that you will be full participants. I sincerely hope that we can work together. And now, can I answer any questions?"

What is the relationship of the skills that make it possible to succeed in academia vs. those that are needed in a leader?

This question is addressed in Chap. 1. Among the skills that are necessary to succeed in the AMC are independence of scholarship in research, novel approaches in clinical work, and originality in teaching and teaching methods/materials. An individual also needs to meet certain criteria for volume, e.g., number of cases or papers and quality measures. None of these necessarily involve teamwork, though they increasingly do. However, each requires at least some separation from the pack, which means being aggressive, competitive, and to some degree self-aggrandizing.

When an individual becomes a leader, however, one goes from being a producer to an enabler. When you are responsible for a division, department, or school, your job is to enable others in your unit to succeed. Accordingly, your focus has to shift from your individual accomplishments to the whole group's success. At a psychological level, you have to shift from feeling good about what you have produced to feeling good about what others have produced (see Chap. 6 on emotional intelligence and other-centeredness and Chap. 15 on recruiting candidates with emotional intelligence).

Skill sets that lead to success as an individual faculty member vs. those required by leaders can be found in some candidates for these jobs, but not all. You need to look for both when you pick your leader.

As an aside, what are your thoughts on the dean's original idea that a superior academic researcher was the way to build a research program?

It is a common perception that to build a research program, you need a person who is a distinguished researcher himself or herself. It's not clear to us that the assumption has been proven to be always correct. There are certainly examples of non-laboratory scientists who have led a great growth in their institution's research portfolio. One view is that building a good research program requires someone who is committed to the idea that research is essential to an outstanding medical school and who has come from an institution where research is a highly valued commodity. But it is actually more the commitment and belief system and knowing how to get it done than the actual time spent in a lab that is important. Understanding this is essential because in the effort to get a proven researcher, there often comes a skill set that is fine for the lab, but not for leadership.

Chapter 15 touches on this same issue with the discussion of the membership of search committees. As we continue to set up committees with constituent groups, we tacitly encourage the members to look for the people who most approximate themselves, on the assumption that they will value what they do. This case shows that the opposite can occur, as it did in this case, because Dr. W didn't respect the work done by members of his department. In fact, he disparaged it and them.

Chapter 28
Negotiating for a Center Director

You are chair of the department of cell biology. You are recruiting for a member of the department in proteomics. The successful candidate has to be not only an outstanding independent investigator but also the director of the proteomic core facility. In fact, the money for the position comes from the proteomic facility and so running that unit is job #1.

So far, one candidate is favored by most of the faculty. She has a history of R01 funding, and in her seminar she was innovative and seen as intellectually ahead of the other candidates.

In your discussions with her, she says she is happy where she is and has put up some big numbers to make it worthwhile for her to move. Her request for lab space exceeds the allotment of others of her rank, and her request for a discretionary fund of $1M (to allegedly make up what monies she would need to leave behind) also exceeds what others of like position have. Otherwise, the number of new positions she would like is available within the package you have, and her equipment requirements are already within the proteomic facility. However, you are getting a bit concerned that she has raised no issues with regard to what would be expected of her in the role of director of the proteomic facility.

You have spoken with colleagues at her home institution. She is uniformly described as bright with a high IQ. Some say she is very direct and gets right in your face in personal debates. One commented that she doesn't suffer fools.

You are thinking she would be fine as a faculty member, but you are not sure how she would be as director of the proteomic facility. The problem is that the package for the proteomic facility came from a donor, and he wants a star in that position.

Negotiating begins with an understanding of the other parties and their interests (and your own interests).

What would you do?

The case in a nutshell is this: this case is included to review the basic concepts of negotiating, particularly positional and issue-oriented negotiating (Chap. 8).

© Springer International Publishing Switzerland 2015   181
J.L. Houpt et al., *Learning to Lead in the Academic Medical Center*,
DOI 10.1007/978-3-319-21260-9_28

The case in Chap. 8, Dr. White, is a much more robust case, so you might want to review it in some detail with the class before discussing this case.

Of all the decisions a leader makes, selection is arguably the most important. "Getting the right people on the bus" is paramount, as Jim Collins noted [1]. The three most common errors in selection are, first, picking a "star" without defining what star means (which leaves one vulnerable to picking skillful, often self-promoting narcissists); second, picking someone in one's own image (thereby amplifying the weaknesses of the leader); or, third, picking someone who is an "expert" (as opposed to an organization-building communicator). In many cases organizations pick experts rather than leaders. A candidate's record of achievements and individual accomplishments can be in important ways irrelevant in identifying and selecting a good leader. In contrast a person with a strong altruistic, team-oriented approach can be an extraordinary leader in situations where there are multiple missions and constituents that need to be motivated and orchestrated.

The way to begin the case discussion is to ask the group to identify the most important elements in an issue-oriented negotiation. Negotiating begins with an understanding of their own and the other parties' interests.

Based on the discussion so far, what are the interests of the recruit and those of the chair?

The candidate's interests appear to be her research program. She wants to stay whole in terms of discretionary funds, and she wants to get the additional positions and full access to the latest equipment. The interests of the chair are to add a scholar and find someone who can manage the proteomic facility. He is particularly interested in someone who can develop procedures that ensure equitable access to the equipment and someone who can mentor younger colleagues.

You can tell that the recruit is a positional negotiator by just listening to her. Every issue she raises is a resource for her research. An issue-oriented negotiator would be talking about her plans for the facility and working on a vision for it and be trying to understand what you want from the facility. This is why you want to listen to a candidate's train of thought without prompting her with too many questions. If you jumped in with a number of questions about the facility, she would likely respond to them, and you would miss that she is not tracking on the facility aspect of the position itself.

What kind of questions can you ask to turn a positional negotiation into an issue-oriented one?

This is covered in detail in Chap. 8. Briefly, you begin with general questions about her goals and aspirations and then lead to more concrete questions about what she is trying to accomplish. In this case, you might just say, "I'm getting an idea of what you are trying to accomplish with your research program, but I'm not clear what your vision for the proteomic facility is."

Is it okay to hire her and hope for the best or should you have a discussion with her before you offer the job?

You could make an argument either way. You could hire her without a discussion, just for the purpose of getting her. If you did, you would be expressing your value of a "star" over equity (Chap. 2, Culture). You need to recognize that if you do, you are getting a great scholar, a star, but not a leader of the proteomic facility. You would anticipate problems after she arrived, but you might prefer to fix them after she is there. You might hope that they might be minimal. You could create an advisory board, or even an executive board, that would oversee the facility. You might even anticipate needing to add another person to administer the facility as her assistant.

Or you could take up the issue before she comes. As we mentioned, having a "spat" on the way in is not all bad, because you learn how the other individual will react. If he or she doesn't handle confrontation well, then you don't need to hire that person. If you have the discussion in advance, you could also put into place an oversight board and an assistant at that time. The huge advantage to doing it before she comes is that you have clarified your expectations of her and can evaluate her performance from day 1. You could include metrics for the facility in her compensation. And you are being honest in your expectations.

Reference

1. Collins J. Good to great. New York: HarperCollins; 2001.

Chapter 29
Dr. Un Settled: Negotiation and Middle-Age Dysphoria

Dr. Un Settled is a tenured associate professor in infectious diseases, and her name has just begun to be circulated as a potential division head candidate at a few well-respected programs. She has been happy in her current position but would like something more. While being successful in maintaining grant support, she feels overwhelmed by the prospect of having to keep doing this for another 20 or more years. She feels the pace is just too much. Also she was recently put on some medical school-wide committees and found herself pleasantly surprised at enjoying thinking at that level. She has always been a mentor and has enjoyed that part of her job. Her current division head has no intention of giving up the job.

Un Settled has a spouse who is a pediatrician in a large practice in town. Fortunately, he has a malpractice tail and could move. She has two children, one who is a senior in high school and going off to college next year and another who is a rising junior in high school.

A friend and colleague of hers in gastroenterology, of similar age and academic progression, was recently offered a division head position at an outstanding institution. He turned it down when his current division head made a retention offer which involved a raise, a travel allowance, a promise to help him achieve center designation, and an initiation of steps for consideration of an early promotion. She'd be happy to find a similar solution.

This is not the first retention offer made recently. In fact, the chair of the department was recently retained with a significant financial package to rebuild the department, when he was a finalist for a dean's position. She hates the idea of interviewing in order to get an offer but believes, as do many others, that currently at least you have to get an outside offer to get what you would like to achieve here.

Un Settled seeks your advice.

How would you advise Dr. Un Settled?

The case in a nutshell is this: we're always a little surprised with how many feel trapped by a need to get an offer from outside in order to move up. They feel anger toward the institution, whereas we think it reflects reality and so it has to be adapted

© Springer International Publishing Switzerland 2015

J.L. Houpt et al., *Learning to Lead in the Academic Medical Center*,
DOI 10.1007/978-3-319-21260-9_29

to. However, we don't confront that initially, but rather we begin by focusing on what one should consider when thinking of taking a leadership job.

There are two issues here. One is Dr. Un Settled and her mid-career crisis, and the second is the culture of the school that requires outside offers to move up. With regard to Un Settled's career aspirations, there are also two issues. One is her place in her maturational/career cycle and whether she can gain pleasure from others' successes (Chap. 6 on The Importance of Emotional Intelligence and Chap. 15). The second is her own existential decision. Though she may wish to see it as a problem with the school's policies, it is not, and she needs to own it as her own problem.

The school's policy can be understood as an expression of Darwinism (see Chap. 2). Darwinians would find this policy intuitive and would expect counter-offers to the "fittest" and, in fact, would probably insist on written proof of offers. Or it could just be a situational factor.

> For a time when I was dean at UNC, deans were evaluated in their five year review on whether they had retained faculty recruited elsewhere. This came about at a time when faculty were being raided largely in the Arts and Sciences campus in response to State cuts. To the business people on the board it seemed like a good strategy. Unfortunately, it had unintended consequences – encouraging the better faculty to get offers and then responding with large counter-offers.

What questions/issues would you want Un Settled to think about in order to help her make her own decision?

You would want her to think about her place in her maturational cycle (Chap. 15) and her stated interest in mentoring to get at the issue of her being able to take pleasure in others' doing well. The idea is to see if her aspirations fit with her maturational age and emotional intelligence. In this case, from what we know, they likely do. If they don't, you need to raise more questions about whether this is a fit for her or just an escape route from writing grants.

The second issue here is her spouse and children. You should see if she has discussed the matter with her husband and where he is as well as the children. One assumes that a rising junior would never want to move, but ask and verify, and see if she plans to move only after that child goes off to college.

This is a life-altering decision. She attributes the cause to the institution's practice of offers and counter-offers. But she needs to separate these issues. Does she want to move up to an administrative decision, and if she were offered one from outside, would she move? Only she can answer this dilemma. Her chair cannot answer it for her. She can seek the boss's assistance after she answers the dilemma for herself. The point here is not to precipitate a negotiation with the chair, particularly one in which the result might be negative, as a way to answer her own dilemma. It's too easy to get the wrong answer that way.

Thus far, we've focused on the personal decision. What about the culture of the institution, which seems to require an outside offer in order to move up? There are many ways to approach this in a class discussion. One is to question whether this is a long-standing practice of the institution or a recent phenomenon. If long standing, then Chap. 2 on Culture Is King and the discussion of Darwinism vs. care and feeding are relevant. In a Darwinian environment, the answer usually is that you may have to go out and get an offer. If this is a recent pattern, there may be other causes. We know of institutions that evaluate their deans on whether they retain or lose faculty, with bonuses tied to retention. This practice establishes an incentive for the dean to try and retain all faculty. In this case, the faculty see multiple retention packages offered, which, in turn, breeds a culture of going outside to get an offer.

You can turn this problem around and ask members of the group how they would want to run things if they were the boss. Would they want a culture of offer and counter-offer? Creating this culture is easy: you just require offers and then try to recruit back. Breaking the cycle is easy, too. If you want to stop people pleading with you for more money, space, etc., once they get an offer, you just let some people go. As soon as it's apparent that you are not going to counter, the behavior stops.

> I didn't want this environment. And I certainly didn't wait until an offer was finally made if I wanted to counter offer. My belief was that if you wait until the person and spouse have spent many dinner conversations on this topic, and made trips to look at houses, they are too far down an emotional road to pull them back. I preferred to make my decision early, as soon as I learned of interest elsewhere, and decide yea or nay about a counter offer at that point.

As far as Un Settled's situation, she needs to determine the prevailing culture. Let's say it's Darwinian. She needs to play by the rules and get an offer, unless she decides that she is just not prepared to do so. As we said earlier, this is a personal existential decision. You need to make it and be comfortable with yourself. This is not a question that others can answer for you.

Let's say Un Settled decides she is not going to move at all, or not unless she absolutely has to, and then only maybe. She decides to talk to her division head. How would you introduce the topic?

In this case you refer to Chap. 8 on Negotiation. This case follows all the same steps as we followed with Dr. White as an entry-level assistant professor. You begin with asking his or her advice on mid-career planning. You emphasize how much you've enjoyed being here and have benefitted by all the opportunities afforded you, but you find your interests changing, and you'd like to see if there is a way to pursue these within the overall goals of the division. You go on to talk of your interest in mentoring and the desire to run a program, like a mini-center focused on a particular topic.

As mentioned in Chap. 11 on Mastering the Art of Persuasion, you pause here and wait for him or her to ask for more. If he or she encourages you to continue, you provide a paragraph on what this center would look like.

Just like in Chap. 8 with Dr. White, who did not mention the man who made more money, you do not mention your friend in GI and the deal he got. Recall that it is too hard to prove that you are the same; that argument is a loser. Also it's the trap of the positional negotiator. Further, you should understand the differences between GI and ID. The GI head probably has more funds with which to make a counter-offer. The ID chief probably does not have surplus funds and so would need to go hat in hand to the chair.

Let's say Un Settled decides to pursue an invitation to interview elsewhere but is still not decided if she really wants to leave. Should she tell her division head and how might she frame that discussion if she did?

The only rule of thumb here is that the division head should hear from you and not from someone else. Thus, you will need to assess the security of the interview process and decide when the right time is to speak with your chair. It's better to be early than late. Search firms do a pretty good job of keeping candidates' names confidential. Faculty search committees often do not do nearly as well. When you meet, it's best to use the meeting as a chance to get mentored/advised. You can explain your desire to go through the process but still indicate your commitment to the current division.

Chapter 30
Dr. Green, Conflict Resolution, and Managing Up and Down

Dr. Green has served six months as chair of surgery. The dean had appointed him as an outside candidate over the strenuous objections of the powerful previous chair, Dr. Black, a vascular surgeon. Dr. Black had lobbied hard, though unsuccessfully, for his protégé in the division of vascular surgery and division chief, Dr. Cole, to succeed him as chair. Dr. Black has been actively undermining Dr. Green's efforts to bring greater harmony to a highly fractured department and to substantially increase revenues and improve a generally anemic research base in the department, all of which he had been charged to do by the dean when he was appointed.

Revenues from vascular surgery in particular are at risk because of intense competition in the surrounding markets. As a solution, the division of vascular surgery, led by Drs. Cole and his mentor, Dr. Black, has been fighting hard to separate themselves from general surgery and to form a separate department of vascular and endovascular surgery. They apparently made a reasonable and legitimate, though not compelling, clinical and business case for doing so. Other divisions are strongly opposed.

The announcement by another prominent medical school in the state that they have created a new department of vascular and endovascular surgery has inflamed the vascular surgery faculty, who are now irate that their already-declining competitive position will be compromised further by the other school's announcement and enhanced visibility. They demand a joint meeting with Dr. Green and the dean.

What would you do?

The case in a nutshell is this: usually, this case arouses the emotions of the group. Mostly, they assail the behavior of Dr. Black and see a threat to Dr. Green's authority. They also question the decision of the dean in bringing Dr. Green into this charged situation in the first place. This permits us to make the most important point in this case. Don't permit the emotion of a situation to become the first consideration.

This case presents three points made in the book. First, based on the algorithm in Chap. 13, forget the emotions for a moment. You can come back to them later.

© Springer International Publishing Switzerland 2015

J.L. Houpt et al., *Learning to Lead in the Academic Medical Center*,

DOI 10.1007/978-3-319-21260-9_30

Instead, ask yourself, what is the best answer to the question of whether vascular services should become independent? What is the business case, and what is the case for teaching and research? What is the effect on the department, the school, and the health system? In "Making Good Decisions," we commented that making decisions based only on political reasons makes you a politician, and on psychological factors alone, a therapist. The job of the leader is to make decisions based on the best interests of the department and institution. We offer the following algorithm: subtract the political and psychological factors to find the ideal solution, and then factor them back in to find the best solution, in these circumstances.

This case also is a reminder that conflict resolution should begin with an exploration of interests. It should be treated like any negotiation. And finally the case provides a context to explore the differences between managing up and managing down.

In this case, the vignette says that a "reasonable and legitimate, though not compelling" case was made. From this we can assume that the business case is a 50/50 deal and that we can turn our attention to the interests of the parties involved.

What are the interests at stake for Dr. Green? For the Department? For the Dean? For Dr. Black?

Every attempt to mediate or work through conflict needs to begin with a question of each party's interests (Chap. 10, Conflict Resolution: Making Friends with Conflict). For Dr. Green his authority is at stake. He is in his first six months where authority is normally bestowed or not (Chap. 3, Authority Is Earned, Not Bestowed, and Chap. 7 on Getting Started the Right Way). The conflict with the former chair has become a public soap opera. Unless Dr. Green handles (wins) this power struggle, he will not be effective in his role.

For the department, its financial future is at stake. But just as importantly, so are its values—most importantly whether a bully (Dr. Black) can prevail. Power struggles could become the way to force his will on people. Will a Darwinian free-for-all prevail, or will laws of civility hold sway (Chap. 2 on Culture Is King)?

For the dean, his authority is also at stake. For reasons we don't know, he chose Dr. Green over Dr. Cole. We also don't know whether the dean hastened Dr. Black's stepping down or not and what their relationship is. It's entirely possible that Dr. Black's behavior in this instance mirrors his behavior earlier and the dean assisted Dr. Black in stepping down.

With regard to Dr. Black, we know his position, but not his interests (see Chap. 8). We know he wanted Dr. Cole to be chair and to have a separate division. While we might assume his motivations and interests, we really don't know them yet.

What would you advise Dr. Green to do?

How does he manage his relationship with the dean?

He tells the dean that while Dr. Black is a pain, he is going to study the merits of the proposal and he has asked some people in the business school to assist him. Getting the imprimatur of the business school is important because he needs his analysis of the business case to be unassailable. He asks the dean to delay the meeting until he has that analysis and he has a chance to talk with some more faculty.

How does he manage his relationship with the other divisions in the department?

He meets with them and tells them that he has asked the business school to assess the business plan and that he wants to fully understand their interests. He meets with them and does a lot of listening.

How does he manage his relationship with vascular surgeons?

Same as above with the other faculty.

How does he manage Dr. Black?

The approach here is the same as with any negotiation (Chap. 8). You can antici- pate that Dr. Black will bombard you with his position, when what you want to know are his interests. You should review the section on the types of questions you might ask to get from positions to interests (Chap. 8). You want to know what inter- ests led to his position to separate vascular surgery. It may only be personality—his narcissism and unwillingness to give up the reins. But there may be some legitimate business reasons, and if there are, there may be the basis of a "win-win" compro- mise. Since the business case is where you have potential openings, you might ask him, "You know, I asked the business school to review the business case. Tell me what you would say to them—how would you make your case."

Let's say that having followed all of these steps, you hear from the business school, and the situation is this. If vascular breaks away from general surgery, they will benefit financially, but the department will do worse. This is because vascular is subsidizing the department's teaching and research mission. Thus, the department will suffer. How would you proceed if you were Dr. Green?

This outcome is typical of what often happens. When you wash away all the drama and emotions, you come down to a conflict between individual self-interest and group (institutional or departmental in this case) interest.

This now becomes an issue for Dr. Green and the dean. Do they want surgery organized as a series of individual units, all on strict financial incentive systems, or do they want the divisions to be interdependent? If they move to independent units, then some of the units will move into the red unless they give up teaching and research and thus will become strictly clinical units. They could go ahead with inde- pendence and give each unit a clear, transparent view of their finances and then impose a tax for education and research. They could each year assess teaching and research and decide what their tax will be. Thus, they could have some measure of independence in terms of bookkeeping and transparency but still support teaching and research. If they go the independence pathway without taxes for research and teaching, they will need a subsidy from somewhere (usually the hospital who ben- efits from their clinical work) or they will need to give up their academic mission. On the other hand, they could remain interdependent and face the possibility of some or all of vascular surgery leaving. The point is that they have clear options based on data, not emotions. It's their call.

In the end, Dr. Green, after consulting with the dean and the hospital and getting input from all parties, has to make a decision. He calls a meeting, reports on the business school analysis, and outlines these options. He needs to take a stand. Not all decisions can be made by consensus. He needs to tell the department what he is going to do and take ownership.

What are the common themes in managing up and down? Where do they diverge?

They both involve letting the faculty know your plans and that you are moving to a solution and how the solution will be reached. When managing up, one must first and foremost not allow surprises. This means early warnings to those above you organizationally about potential collateral damage. Managing down emphasizes the involvement of the faculty and their part in the solution to the crisis.

> It took me many years to learn that communication wasn't what I said to the faculty, but what they said to me. When they're talking, I'm communicating.

Chapter 31
Drs. Rich and Pure: Conflict of Interest (COI) and Creating School-Wide Policies

In the past decade, the power within the department of medicine has resided in the division of cardiology. The division is heavily involved in industry-funded clinical trials as well as clinical care. The division's faculty has extensive ties with industry, including lucrative speaking engagements, training programs for other cardiologists, particularly in the procedural subspecialties, and three start-up companies built around various cardiac devices invented by division faculty along with surgery faculty. NIH funding for the department has declined in the past three years but is still relatively strong in relation to other departments of medicine nationally.

Last year, there was a scandal within the cardiology division that reverberated through the school and university. It involved a nationally prominent professor in the cardiology division, Dr. Rich, with large, active NIH grants, who failed to report on his annual conflicts of interest disclosure $500,000 in consulting fees from speaking engagements at a major pharma company. His NIH grants involve two compounds in which the company is interested. The fallout from NIH was serious.

Dr. Pure, also a professor in the division, has written extensively on the topic of physician/industry relationships, arguing that there should be no personal financial interests with industry and no CME funding from industry. He has a strong following among the fellows and students but not among other faculty. The local papers as well as the national press have editorialized on the subject of pharma and device companies buying prominent figures in academic medicine. The university's Board of Trustees has demanded that conflicts of interest be cleaned up. At the same time, they have urged the university administration to aggressively pursue industry funding of research as well as industry gifts for the university's new capital campaign.

There is a new dean of the school who has been in place for six months. She has brought you in as the new chair of medicine from a private institution, where you were chief of cardiology. She wants you to lead the effort to clean up the relationships with industry, but she is conscious of the need to retain strong, nationally prominent faculty and good relationships with industry (the source of increasing industry support for clinical trials). Ideally, she wants you to "cinch down," school-wide, on personal relationships with industry while keeping everybody happy.

© Springer International Publishing Switzerland 2015
J.L. Houpt et al., *Learning to Lead in the Academic Medical Center*,
DOI 10.1007/978-3-319-21260-9_31

She would like for you to enlist the support of other chairs so that the effort can be made to "stick" school-wide.

What would you do?

The case in a nutshell is this: our classes often start by diving into the COI questions. There seems to be no shortage of opinions. That's okay, but the case is a two-step one. First, there's the question of the policy, but also we have to get the policy implemented. So that's where we start.

COI is a charged issue, and people often hold passionate but opposite views. It's also an important issue because it strikes at some basic values regarding professionalism. The case is complicated by the fact that the chair is new and thus hasn't yet been bestowed his or her authority. The solution is going to require even more listening than normal because of the chair's novice status. Finally, this case requires dealing with a large array of characters—trustees, dean, chairs, division heads, polarizing people (Rich and Pure), students, and house staff—so the ideas in Chap. 14 on Simulating Change Without Enduring a Coup are highly relevant, and you need to develop a strategy to deal with the various parties.

Where would you start?

Before you leap into the question of how to manage all these moving parts, you'd be wise to sit down with a piece of paper and list the known parameters of the case—both the knowns and the unknowns. This is an effort to force you to be strategic and limit the field of play.

Why me? Why was I chosen to lead this effort? This is the first unknown. Usually, a dean would select an established and respected member of the community (village elder) to lead such an effort. But you were chosen probably to bring an outside voice and because your department is the main player in this drama.

Yet you are new to the institution, without the necessary credibility to "make this stick" on your own.

Unless you are just being thrown to the wolves, your choice to lead this effort probably reflects the confidence and high opinion that the dean has of you. Even so, you need to think about how to make up for being a new and unknown entity.

> I was in a similar situation when I was at Emory. I was the newest and least experienced chair when the new dean asked me to lead a committee on the future of the school at Grady Hospital. It was a charged situation, and the existing chairs were not pleased that one of them was not leading this effort, because as I learned they had very strong opinions that were contrary to those of the dean. In this case I was being thrown to the wolves, whereas in the one above, the dean most likely wanted you to lead it because cardiology was the biggest player. I faced the same issue of credibility and concluded early that any recommendation would require the chairs' agreement. Given these circumstances, I limited the committee to just the other major clinical chairs and met until we had a common sense of what we wanted to do.

The "why me" question leads directly to the second question, "who should be on the committee." One way to start is to decide that this committee has to have the necessary power people on it, in order to build buy-in, so that they can sell the outcome to their constituencies. The idea is to use their credibility. This is difficult for some people because they assume that their title buys them credibility, but it doesn't.

It has to be earned (Chap. 3), so in this case you acquire it by using the already-earned credibility of others.

Since this is to be "school-wide," the committee has to broader than the chairs. There needs to be a resident and probably a residency training director. Then there is the question of whether a trustee should be on the committee. When we discuss this in our classes, there is usually a disagreement here. Some think a trustee should not be on the committee. They think that the trustees should receive the report, be informed as the committee proceeds, but the presence in the room of a trustee representative might bring too much influence to bear. Others would add the trustee, with the chancellor's approval, to make sure that the solution meets the trustees' expectations. The argument here is that you have a big problem if you get consensus and buy-in, and the trustees reject it at their level. That would not make for a happy dean. In the classes, we acknowledge that either would work as long as the trustees are informed. Finally, you'd look for village elders. The question of whether Dr. Rich or Pure should be on the committee is dealt with below.

The third question is "what really is our task." This is a known. Much has already been decided. The trustees and dean have already decided that we will have relationships with industry. Thus, the tussle between Drs. Pure and Rich, while entertaining drama, is really irrelevant to the discussion. Dr. Pure loses because there will be financial ties to industry, although his CME question is still up for consideration. And Dr. Rich loses because, of course, there will need to be disclosure.

Narrowing the field of debate is important to winning any debate. If you open the question of whether we should have relationships with industry, you have opened Pandora's box. People who can stimulate change and get hard things done constantly narrow the field of dispute. In this case, the trustees answered that larger question of whether or not there should be such relationships.

The fourth question is what the best practices are in this area. This is also a known. The question to the committee has been narrowed to how we can relate to industry in a way that minimizes conflict of interest or intent. There are several monographs and excellent policies at other places on the topic, and they should be made available to the committee.

Getting things done and being a successful change agent requires these steps in terms of policy as much as if not more than effort is spent on implementation. This is a hard lesson for many to learn, which is why so many white papers collect dust rather than being implemented. This point is detailed in Chap. 14 on Stimulating Change Without Enduring a Coup.

Develop a strategy for dealing with the dean.

You review with her your conclusions from the four questions above. You ask if she agrees, sees problems with them, or wants to ask anything. You ask her view on the trustee member of the committee—whether it is a good idea, and if so, who it should be. If she likes the idea, you ask her to invite the trustee to be on the committee.

Develop a strategy for dealing with the faculty of the division, including Dr. Rich and Dr. Pure.

You need to decide if you will have a member of the division on the committee or not. A lot will depend on whether there is a relatively neutral voice who has not sided with Drs. Rich and Pure. And since you are emphasizing the school-wide nature of this, there may be some asymmetry with only one division head and all other chairs. You also need to guarantee to keep the faculty informed and permit them to speak to the committee. You would explain the limited charge—that you are not determining whether there will be relationships with industry but rather how they should be structured to minimize COIs.

And what should you do with Dr. Rich and Pure—include them on the committee or not? Our groups divide over this issue as well. It opens a good discussion on when to put adversaries/polarizing figures into the tent and when to put them outside the tent. There is no single answer here.

I favor not putting them on the committee for two reasons. First, I don't want this to be about them. It is merely a discussion of best practices. Second, if they are on the committee, and they draw some support, the committee will develop a "plank" for them, much like a political convention. In the end, you'll have a solution with some "pork" for them and possibly every other constituency.

Develop a strategy for dealing with the fellows and the students.

The same as above, repeat the narrowed charge and announce that they will be represented.

Develop a strategy for dealing with the other chairs.

You meet with them and spend some time explaining the narrow charge and seeking their input. This is your power base. You spend as much time as is necessary to get their intellectual and emotional buy-in. As stated above, when all is done, they will make it work or not. You meet with them separately before convening the large committee.

If this process works correctly, it should end with a whimper rather than a bang. By that we mean that the chairs in particular will buy into it, and because they will be the ones to enforce the policy, it will be implemented.

It shouldn't happen, but what if the committee looking at this becomes hopelessly deadlocked and can't come to consensus? What do you do?

As a dean, I have been in this situation a few times. Each side is genuinely opposed to the other view and win-wins are not possible. Usually, in these cases, there is an emotional attachment to an ideal or value that is sacrosanct, or there is a commitment to a person who is a central figure in the conflict and loyalty prevails.

I have found only one way out of it. The most important step is to take a stand yourself. It may be with the majority or minority – it doesn't matter. The second step is to acknowledge that there can be no agreement reached – kind of like a "hung jury" – and that you favor issuing a majority and minority report. If that occurred in this example, you would meet with the dean and trustee and explain to them why there will be no agreement within the group. You tell them also your opinion. They can disband the group or they can have you present a majority and minority report, and then can make their own decision that then becomes policy.

Chapter 32
Budget Cuts and Managing Bad News and Incentivizing

You are the new chair of a clinical department in the medical school. One of your initial efforts is to create a departmental compensation plan. You create a task force, which works for nearly a year on a new plan, balancing out appropriate rewards for clinical, research, and other mission-related productivity. The plan includes a baseline salary, which is to be the median salary for that specialty, role (clinical versus research), and rank based on national data from the prior three years. An incentive plan includes payments for RVUs generated in excess of the median benchmark, along with incentives for funding of research effort and other mission/citizenship work. In the end, there is enthusiasm for the plan because many faculty will see increases in salary, as faculty below national means will see annual raises of the maximum allowable percent until their salaries reach the appropriate level. For some faculty, this would require 3–5 years of annual raises, given that current salaries are so low.

Less than one year later, the state cuts funding to the School of Medicine (SOM). The dean sends an email to all the departments and faculty. In it he says that the SOM must reduce its expenditures by $8M to accommodate the decrease in state funding. He points out that there will be personnel and non-personnel expense reductions in the dean's office and encourages departments to do the same. He sends out specific expense reduction targets by department.

Since this memo was sent from the dean's office to the entire faculty, you quickly learn that the following attitudes and concerns are right on the surface with the faculty:

1. Several members of the department have undergone nonrenewals of their contracts in the last 5 years, including faculty who were perceived by their peers to have done good work. This caused significant problems with overall departmental morale at the time, and those effects are still lingering. Additionally, fixed-term faculty are beginning to wonder if they too are at risk.
2. Other faculty members are counting on the raises that were promised to them as part of the faculty compensation plan. Although the fine print of the plan states

© Springer International Publishing Switzerland 2015   197
J.L. Houpt et al., *Learning to Lead in the Academic Medical Center*,
DOI 10.1007/978-3-319-21260-9_32

that its implementation is contingent on state funding, the faculty heard you promise raises.

3. Your faculty note that the memo from the dean addresses only reduction of expenses, not increasing revenue. They argue that reducing the numbers of faculty members will reduce income, which is a goal seemingly contradictory to the vision of the department (and the reason you were hired) to stimulate growth. Reducing support staff will decrease efficiency and therefore also reduce productivity, income, and growth. They want you to go to the dean and argue against expense reduction in favor of revenue generation.

You also meet with the dean's budget people and with your own and find out that your department's share of the cuts is 3 % of your personnel budget, which, together with the 6 % increase in budget that was necessary to get all the pay raises accomplished, gives you a new 9 % hole.

How would you think through this dilemma and determine your cuts and how would you communicate it to the faculty?

What would you do?

The case in a nutshell is this: this scenario is about delivering bad news. We cover this in Chap. 14, Stimulating Change Without Enduring a Coup. In that chapter, we comment on the need to offer hope and a compelling plan and to move the group from the position of victim to that of activist. The case illustrates that to accomplish this, you must listen to the dissent, and from those concerns find a plan that permits the group's survival but also addresses their values. In any change agenda, values must be addressed. In terms of listening to their dissatisfaction, you need to listen and then present a plan that indicates that you understand what they've said. You don't have to give them everything, but you do need to give them something.

Here are some things to consider:

The primary role of the leader is to protect the group. Can you find a plan that protects the group?

You know that the group wants you to protect them, but there are a limited number of options. One, you can delay the promises of pay raises, give 3 % cuts to all, and promise to start when the financial picture brightens. Or two, you can make cuts of 9 % and thus honor the promise to get compensation up with what you take from the cuts. This will mean cutting people, though some of the cuts could come out of the non-personnel budget. Or three, you could offer some combination of the two—make some progress but not get to where you want to be. In order to assess the merits of each plan, you need to have your business manager get you the details of how much would need to be cut.

In the meantime, you decide to seek the counsel of the village elders. You learn that there have been many attempts to get the salaries up in the past. Efforts failed, often for the same reasons you are facing now. Each time there was an effort, the legislature cut the budget or only allowed a 1 % increase when just the cost of living increase would have produced more. Each time, clinical funds could have been used to bolster the clinicians, but when the legislature insisted on only 1 % raises for those paid from state funds, the department decided out of a sense of equity that everyone (staff and clinicians) should limit themselves to 1 %. Whereas faculty could draw from clinical revenues, the state-funded staff were limited to state-mandated increases.

You begin to understand that this scenario is going to repeat itself and that the issue is not only money but a long-held value of equity—all are treated alike, independent of station and contribution. Whatever plan is put in place will need to address values as well as the financial solution. In this case, there is a conflict between equity and your desire for meritocracy.

This is a lesson learned over and over in the AMC. When something looks like a money issue, it turns out to be a value proposition as well. Or when something looks like a value proposition, it turns out to be personality or money issue. You only learn this by listening and by establishing lines of communication up and down.

Do you separate yourself from the dean and blame him or do you assume that you have to support him with the group?

If a dean is unpopular, there is a tendency to separate yourself from him and act as if you're helpless before his demands. In fact, one reason why vertical hierarchies are as ineffective as they are (see Chap. 1) is that those who are one step below rarely want to use up their social capital on the higher-up's causes.

The problem with the blame game is that it comes back to bite you. If you use blame, your faculty will emulate your behavior and then blame you for everything that harms them. In this case, the dean's letter is pretty straightforward and transparent. He has made his cuts and now it's time for yours. In our thinking, you are wise to support him within your group.

The group wants you to argue with the dean over the expense reduction strategy. Do you do that?

We argue for strategies to enlarge the pie (Chap. 8). But generating revenues is not usually a quick fix, as new programs take time to produce return on investment. The quickest and surest way to adapt to decreased revenue is budget cuts. You are wise here not to bother with this argument. You would only look obstructionist. If there are ways to generate revenues, put them in next year's budget.

This request from the group could be viewed as their need to have you to protect them. A common first reaction is to go fight the one who brought the bad news. You should resist this impulse but meet their needs for protection by finding a solution to the problem.

Should you and your office share in the cuts?

Yes, the dean did and you should as a way to model good behavior.

The finance people outline a plan that is doable even though it involves losing some more fixed-term faculty. Let's say you decide that you want to proceed with it based on **all the information now at your disposal. How do you frame your argument?**

You meet with the village elders and tell them that you feel that you need to move forward because, based on the history, "If we don't do it now, we will always find a reason not to." You believe that the department's commitment to equity is admirable, but over the years, because of inconsistent state support, that value has led to a serious situation that threatens the survival of the group, that is, their inability to keep compensation at market rates. From a departmental point of view, a strong faculty should be the first priority; students come to study with the best faculty and patients get the best care from the best faculty. Staff people are valuable, but their salaries come from the state, and they get paid according to those scales. You can advocate for them and you will, but you hurt the department by keeping compensation in line with staff when you don't have to.

You go on to say that you are taking as much money as you can from non-personnel funds, so you can lighten the blow on fixed-term faculty. You then pause and ask for your faculty's thoughts. After some discussion, they say that they agree with your reasoning but warn you that some will oppose it. You ask for their support and go forward.

Chapter 33
A "No-Brainer": Dr. Virtue Comes to State University Medical Center

Dr. Virtue (Dr. V) has recently been appointed to be the new chair of the department of medicine at State University Medical Center (SUMC). He was brought in from outside, having served as the vice chair of his previous department. Shortly after arriving, he was approached by Associate Dean Dr. Do Good with a request to help sponsor an initiative called "The Code of Conduct." The "Code" is a set of rules or principles designed to promote positive collegial relationships across the medical center. This initiative came about because of several reported incidents of bullying and harassment in the institution. The other driver of this initiative was the most recent physician satisfaction scores from SUMC. The survey measures physician engagement and their perceived quality of work life and collegiality. SUMC placed in the bottom quartile of this national survey.

The Code of Conduct was designed to serve as a set of operating principles to address the problem of what was increasingly described as a hostile work environment and to ensure that people treat one another with respect, refrain from any abusive or intimidating behavior, and promote a positive culture of cooperation. Dr. V was very positive about this initiative. In addition, his prior institution had enacted a similar program called "Rules of the Road," which provided a set of detailed guidelines as a code of conduct.

Dr. V began to champion the program immediately. At one of his first faculty meetings, Dr. V asked the Associate Dean Do Good to present this initiative and field questions the faculty might have. Dr. V was somewhat surprised at the lack of positive reception on the part of his colleagues and the lack of any discussion after Dr. Do Good's presentation. Nevertheless, he proceeded with his plan and appointed a committee (the Culture Taskforce) of respected senior faculty to take the Code, customize it for the department of medicine, and plan how to implement its use as a tool for faculty, staff, and student performance evaluations. While he had some difficulty getting some of the physicians to agree to serve on the task force, he attributed their reluctance to the usual challenge of getting busy physicians to engage in service activities. Dr. V was convinced that this initiative would support his broader objective of making the department of medicine a center of excellence, distinguished

© Springer International Publishing Switzerland 2015   201
J.L. Houpt et al., *Learning to Lead in the Academic Medical Center*,
DOI 10.1007/978-3-319-21260-9_33

by its positive culture and productive work environment for research, teaching, and clinical service.

Six months later, when Dr. V is in his sixth month of tenure as department chair, he sees clear signs of progress in some areas, but he is disturbed by a lack of progress in his efforts to develop a more positive departmental culture. He was realistic, he thought, about the likelihood of some resistance, but he did not expect the overt challenge and hostility communicated by his colleagues (particularly ones who he had seen as his support base). He knew there was a lot of behind-the-scenes talk among senior faculty about being on a "forced march," which was part of a larger backlash against what many faculty saw as the imposition of a business-driven corporate culture.

As Dr. V was to learn, the backlash was a response to SUMC's top management's efforts to bring business practices and discipline to the AMC. The CEO of SUMC Healthcare and her high-level administrators brought a different bottom-line-oriented perspective to the institution. They communicated a clear message about efficiency, cutting costs, and generating revenue. This message was followed by the administration's strong efforts to enforce compliance with new metrics and processes designed to make financial management and discipline the order of the day.

After several members of the Culture Taskforce had resigned in protest over what they saw as yet another example of being "corporatized" *and* infantilized ("telling us how to behave"), Dr. V had to appoint some junior (but tenured) faculty. They were more supportive of the effort, and on a number of key issues they moved things forward for a while by outvoting their senior colleagues. This led to thinly veiled threats by their senior colleagues and protests about the "tyranny of the majority." As the rancor increased, the younger faculty members' support for the Code began to waver. At this point, Dr. V muses, the net effect of the culture change effort is negative—it has spawned a divisive, adversarial backlash that threatens to undermine every cooperative initiative he wants to initiate in the department.

Dr. V has no idea what to do to get his efforts on track. He wonders why a program of such obvious importance and value flounders so badly. What should he have done to prevent this adverse outcome? How could he have anticipated this reaction? What can he do to turn things around?

What Would You Do?

This Is the Case in a Nutshell Let the group talk about this from any angle they wish. You are just trying to gauge their hostility or acceptance of the recent changes to a "corporate model" as described in this case.

While we know that thinking like a leader requires a person to rise above partisan politics and take on a more statesmanlike role, it is not always clear what that means in a specific situation, especially where the contending factions generate conflict and dissent. A leader caught in the middle between two sides can understandably feel divided with the resulting desire to keep each of the conflicting parties happy—in this case, those promoting the new values initiative vs. those wanting to drop the whole values initiative effort. This either/or thinking leaves a leader in an untenable and unmanageable situation.

Fortunately, there is a way forward. Thinking like a leader involves moving from either/or reasoning to both/and analysis. This involves trying to understand issues not as problems to be resolved but as polarities that require balancing. Many situations that leaders face appear to be either/or choices (i.e., short-term vs. long-term performance, centralized vs. decentralized control, traditional approaches vs. innovative ones) that need to be "resolved." In reality these ongoing normative tensions require balancing, not solving or resolving, as if they were a problem with a solution.

Think of the dichotomous values outlined in Chap. 2, Culture is King. In this case, the leader needs to respect the traditional values of the academic institution (autonomy) while promoting new ways of coordinating and collaborating (shared values) to compete in a changing healthcare environment. In this context, the leader has to help both sides see the value of the other side so that traditional ways of operating that are still viable are respected and preserved, while new ways of managing (using shared values and enhanced teamwork) can be embraced to sustain the organization's success [1, 2].

What sense can you make of this if you analyze what happened from the point of view of a top-down management style that utilizes a vertical hierarchy to stimulate change and where the senior faculty are disaffected village elders?

Looked at this way, the reaction makes sense and is no longer a no-brainer. As outlined in Chap. 1, top-down tactics often don't work because there is no guaranteed buy-in. In this case, we have the proverbial "last straw" syndrome where the faculty finally say they've had enough—that's it. "We run the place," they say. And sure enough, as village elders, they do, even if the corporate administrators think they do. So the village elders heap enough displeasure on the junior faculty and the junior faculty fold.

Dr. Virtue should never have been surprised. He should know that faculty look on what they view as corporate intrusions into their autonomy as violations of their academic freedom and professionalism. Younger faculty are not as sensitive since they never have known or enjoyed the unfettered freedom that older faculty have enjoyed.

Recall the case of Dr. Rose (Chaps. 16 and 25). He also was naïve. In both cases, being naïve brings problems because the group concludes that you cannot protect them. If Dr. Virtue had anticipated their potential displeasure and just asked them for their thoughts, he wouldn't have looked naïve because he knew to ask. Further, he might have nipped this whole rebellion on the bud.

How Can He Turn This Around?

He needs to get his faculty to see that this "corporate take-over," specifically, the Code of Conduct, is harmless and doesn't really take any more autonomy away. While they are casting it as autonomy vs. corporate dictates, it is in reality only an attempt to articulate some shared values and build a community of collegiality. He should point out the value that they, as senior citizens, could bring to that effort. He needs to understand their frustration but needs to find other ways for them to channel it. He could simply sit down with them and say, "Let's talk about all the changes in the last few years that have led to your disaffection, and let's see if we can come up with some things that will make your life more satisfying." In this way, he would be moving from either/or to both/and.

To Teachers You may want to then ask the class to anticipate the future of the AMC, using this vignette, as a lead-in to this important topic. What is viewed here as corporate influence—treatment pathways, guidelines, metrics, and more top-down engineering—is unlikely to change. Ask what they think of it and what they might do.

References

1. Martin R. How successful leaders think. Boston: Harvard Business Review; 2007.
2. Johnson B. Polarity management, identifying and managing unsolvable problems. Amherst: HRD Press Inc.; 1996.

Appendix A
Developmental Steps

1. Recognizing strengths as potential liabilities is an example of a general need for AMC leaders to develop the capacity for counter-intuitive thinking;
2. Learning to leverage yourself, developing high levels of discipline around delegation and empowerment (working smarter, not harder, which is often counter-intuitive for successful people);
3. Learning to live with higher degrees of uncertainty and ambiguity in a complex system;
4. Dealing with personal and, we hope, temporary incompetence as you, the leader, learn new roles and master new situations;
5. Giving up your role as an individual contributor to become a team member and/ or team leader;
6. Learning to be fully competent by creating informal alliances and partnerships with people who are more competent than you are in critical areas (e.g., legal, financial, operations, information systems, lobbying, and development);
7. Learning to deal with a much broader range of constituents both inside and outside the AMC, many of whom have greater seniority, visibility, and power than you;
8. Learning to deal with new, complex and sometimes invisible constituencies;
9. Learning to manage higher levels of conflict at institutional levels;
10. Dealing with the power of the media and its impact on all of your constituents;
11. Learning to understand the impact of your own personality and style on the culture and performance of a very political environment, often with limited or unreliable feedback;
12. Developing a set of trusted advisors at multiple levels of the organization to give you direct and candid feedback and counsel;
13. Mastering emotional currents, an under-recognized force in academic settings where ideas and reason serve as the official currency of exchange;
14. Transitioning from being a steward of institutional values to becoming a visible advocate and spokesperson in an environment of competing values;

© Springer International Publishing Switzerland 2015
J.L. Houpt et al., *Learning to Lead in the Academic Medical Center*,
DOI 10.1007/978-3-319-21260-9

15. Becoming responsible for enhancing and sustaining an environment where everyone can achieve their potential in their respective jobs and their roles as managers and leaders;
16. Learning to build broad coalitions to take action—although you may climb to the top of a formal organization with one set of skills, a very different set of skills may be required to manage the informal organization, which has the capacity to determine your ultimate success;
17. Creating a vision or at least a shared sense of direction and focus for those around you; and
18. Finding balance between the demands of work, especially evening and weekend obligations, and your physical and emotional wellbeing.

Appendix B
Questions on Interpersonal and Management Skills

Interpersonal

- Understands a person's feelings and the concerns behind those feelings;
- Can incorporate those concerns into his/her plan of action;
- Understands political realities and creates action plans that take those into account;
- Listens well;
- Asks pertinent questions;
- Offers positive feedback when appropriate;
- Finds opportunity in challenges rather than exhibiting fear or anxiety;
- Can persuasively make a point and sell his/her point of view;
- Can communicate with people of different rank and backgrounds within the department;
- Seizes opportunity;
- Uses the institutions values in developing his/her plans;
- Controls emotions and mood—neither drawn to anger nor inappropriately up or down;
- Evaluates various options without undue bias;
- In all actions he/she has the institution's best interests at heart;
- Makes you proud to be part of this institution.

Management

- Keeps people informed of appropriate issues;
- Gives clear direction;
- Offers advice on how to approach a difficult situation;
- Starts and ends meetings on time;

© Springer International Publishing Switzerland 2015
J.L. Houpt et al., *Learning to Lead in the Academic Medical Center*,
DOI 10.1007/978-3-319-21260-9

- Avoids distractions and keeps focused on the problem;
- Sums up after a group meeting and makes sure everyone knows their assignment;
- Manages his/her time;
- Can set priorities;
- In running meetings, forces discussion to move along without drifting off or moving into diversions or repetitions;
- Can communicate his/her vision;
- Can offer corrective advice in an appropriate way.

Appendix C
Annotated Bibliography

1. "Leadership that gets results," Daniel Goleman, Harvard Business Review, March–April 2000.

   If you read only one leadership article this year, this classic HBR article is the one to read. It describes the links between leadership, emotional intelligence, and organizational climate and performance.

2. What Makes a Leader? Daniel Goleman, Harvard Business Review, November–December, 1998.

   This article describes the five key components of emotional intelligence (EI) at work and addresses the issue of how leaders can improve their level of EI persistence, practice, and reflection.

3. "Leading With Questions: How Leaders Find the Right Solutions by Knowing What to Ask," Michael J. Marquardt, San Francisco, Jossey-Bass, 2005.

   Peter Drucker, the founding father of American management and leadership theory, once commented, "In the past the leader was the person who came up with the right answers, in the future the leader will be the person who comes up with the right questions." This book is a how-to guide designed to help leaders become proficient at asking the right questions at the right time.

   Overcoming these barriers is highly rewarded; leaders who are able to create a "culture of questioning" enhance the prospect for success by:

   (a) Increasing flow of information
   (b) Increasing collaboration and questioning
   (c) Capturing and sharing learning
   (d) Nurturing Innovation
   (e) Establishing sense of urgency

   Finally Marquardt describes different kinds of questions and how to develop your skills in choosing which ones to use based on the situation or problem you are trying to resolve.

© Springer International Publishing Switzerland 2015
J.L. Houpt et al., *Learning to Lead in the Academic Medical Center*,
DOI 10.1007/978-3-319-21260-9

4. "How Managers Become Leaders: The seven seismic shifts in responsibility and perspective," Michael D. Watkins, Boston, Harvard Business Review, June 2012.

This article describes the seven key transitions that leaders must make to become fully developed leaders. They include making the transition from: Specialist to Generalist, Analyst to Integrator, Tactician to Strategist, Bricklayer to Architect, Problem Solver to Agenda Setter, Warrior to Diplomat, and Supporting Cast Member to Lead Role.

Watkins has provided a powerfully descriptive account of the multiple transitions physician managers need to make to become effective leaders. In that context the article provides both a self-assessment tool for appraising one's progress as an individual and an equally useful tool for assessing the emerging capabilities of developing physician leaders.

5. "Building the Emotional Intelligence of Groups," Vanessa Urch Druskat & Steven B. Wolff, Harvard Business Review, March 2001.

Druskat and Wolff provide a very practical model of team effectiveness that can then be put into practice by addressing three levels of group emotional effectiveness (individual, group, and cross boundary). They provide examples of specific norms related to the three levels that a team can address to improve their performance by enhancing the relationships among their members.

6. "What to Ask the Person in the Mirror," Robert S. Kaplan, Harvard Business Review.

Knowing what to ask yourself may be the most important question a leader can ask. In building self-awareness, discipline, and effectiveness the senior leader needs to ask about his or her performance in all of these key areas: vision and priorities, managing time, feedback (giving and receiving), succession planning, evaluation and alignment, leading under pressure, and staying true to oneself. Using these metrics to evaluate and develop yourself can contribute immeasurably to both career success and satisfaction.

7. "The First 90 Days: Critical success strategies for new leaders at all levels," Michael Watkins, Boston, Harvard Business School Press, 2003.

It is typical for senior executives to receive a formal review of their progress in the first 90 days of being in a new job. This article describes the perils and pitfalls of entering into high level responsibilities and provides very clear guidelines about what to pay attention to in order to avoid failures and enhance both short-term and long-term success in a new job with high visibility and risks.

8. "Managing your Boss," John J. Gabarro & John P. Kotter, Harvard Business Review, May–June 1993.

This classic article addresses the challenge that leaders face in exerting power and influence upwards in dealing with their own bosses (or boards). It provides a protocol for understanding the issues and agendas that bosses have to deal with and clear guidance in how to address them to be effective in formal organizational structures. It also provides a clear checklist to help one manage those above them competently.

9. "How Successful Leaders Think," Roger Martin, Harvard Business Review, June 2007.

Roger Martin describes one of the most important but least understood aspects of effective leadership—how leaders think. His compelling observation about how the most competent leaders are able to synthesize conflicting ideas and possibilities to achieve higher-level results is informative, useful, and groundbreaking. Martin provides a simple model to describe the difference between conventional and integrative thinking, which is a crucial insight for leaders to understand if they are to succeed at the highest levels.

10. "Building Your Company's Vision," James C. Collins & Jerry I. Porras, Harvard Business Review, September–October 1996.

Based on their research on America's most successful corporations published in their book, *Built to Last*, the authors examine the roles played by the leaders of these organizations. A key finding is that these leaders were able to balance and integrate the conflicting pulls of constancy and change to create optimal performance and sustainable success. They argue that the most important issue is to understand what changes seldom, if ever, which is purpose (what you offer the world) and values (what you stand for). Holding these constant creates the necessary stability to then support vigorous innovation in products, process and policies so that the organization can offer the most desirable products and services to achieve sustainable high performance.

Index

© Springer International Publishing Switzerland 2015
J.L. Houpt et al., *Learning to Lead in the Academic Medical Center*,
DOI 10.1007/978-3-319-21260-9

Meetings
    conflict areas, diminishing, 108
    group leader, 109–110
    influence groups, 110
    irrational groups, 107
    leader, fundamental task, 108
    negative responses, 107
    on task and on time, groups, 108–109
    weasel, 111
Mental schemas simplification, 5–6
Metaphor, 62, 105
Mission subsidies, 21, 67, 191
Mistakes, 46, 61–63, 67, 86, 101, 116
Mole, 111
Myers–Briggs, 37–39, 43, 53, 178

N
Narcissism, 175
    AMC leaders, 45
    behavior patterns, 47
    emotional card, 48
    institution, 46
    passive aggression, 89
    personalities, 46
    personality disorders, 92
    rage, 48
Negotiation
    BATNA, 77, 78
    cell biology, 181
    commitment, 188
    compensation, 69
    Darwinism, 186
    decision making, 186–187
    demeanor, 78–79
    discretionary fund, 181
    EI, 186
    executive board, 183
    gastroenterology, 185
    infectious diseases, 185
    interests (*see* Interests, negotiation)
    interview process, 188
    issue-orientation (*see* Issue-orientation, negotiation)
    maturational cycle, 186
    mentoring, 187
    mid-career planning, 187
    middle-age dysphoria, 153
    organization-building, 182
    personality factors, 114
    positional, 69, 70
    proteomic facility, 181
    recruitment, 81–87
    relationship, maintaining, 69, 71
    research program, 182
    resources, 135
    school-wide committees, 185
    silence, 78
    start-up package, 69
    successful negotiation, steps, 76–77
    ZOPA, 78

O
On task, 108–109
On time, 108–109
Optimal performance, 128, 211
Organization
    AMC, 3–5
    compensation, 8
    creative *vs.* efficient society, 9–10
    culture, 8–9
    hierarchical systems, 7
    mental schemas simplification, 5–6
Organizational structures, 210

P
Page, 101–102
Paragraph, 101–102
Passive–aggressive personality, 49
Perfectionism, 41, 42, 49–50, 115, 132, 178
Personality
    apology, 179
    compensation plan, 173
    decisions, 186
    EI, 180
    great success, 177
    interpersonal skills, 178
    Myers–Briggs, 178
    narcissism, 178
    national organizations, 179
    NIH presence, 177
    passive–aggressive response, 173
    and political factors, 113
    psychological capacity, 178
    research program, 180
    social niceties, 177
    teaching methods/materials, 179
    traits and leadership, 178
Personality disorders
    narcissism, 45–48
    passive–aggressive personality, 49
    perfectionistic personality, 49–50
Personality traits
    administrative hierarchy, 42–43
    agreeableness, 38
    biographical approaches, 37

CPI Antony Rowe
Eastbourne, UK
March 07, 2019